LIFE OF A BARBER
THE DOS & TABOOS

LIFE OF A BARBER
THE DOs & TABOOs

The Biography of John Tenuta

Gerry Mueller, M.M.C.

Library of Congress Control Number: 2011911339
ISBN: Hardcover   978-1-4628-9473-4
                 Softcover   978-1-4628-9472-7
                 Ebook   978-1-4628-9474-1

To order additional copies of this book, contact:
Xlibris Corporation
1-888-795-4274
www.Xlibris.com
Orders@Xlibris.com
98351

CONTENTS

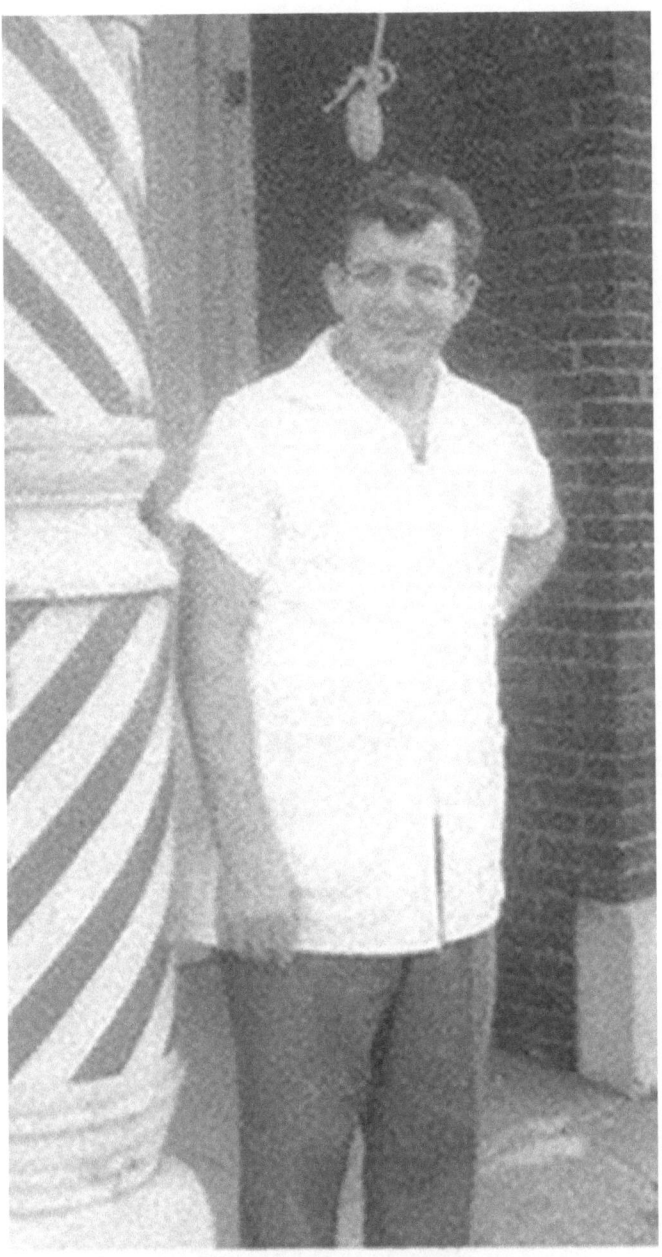

This is John Tenuta at 27 years old standing in front of his his new Cicero Avenue barber shop wearing a jacket made by his mother-in law, Adelina.

DESCENDANTS OF ANGELO TENUTA

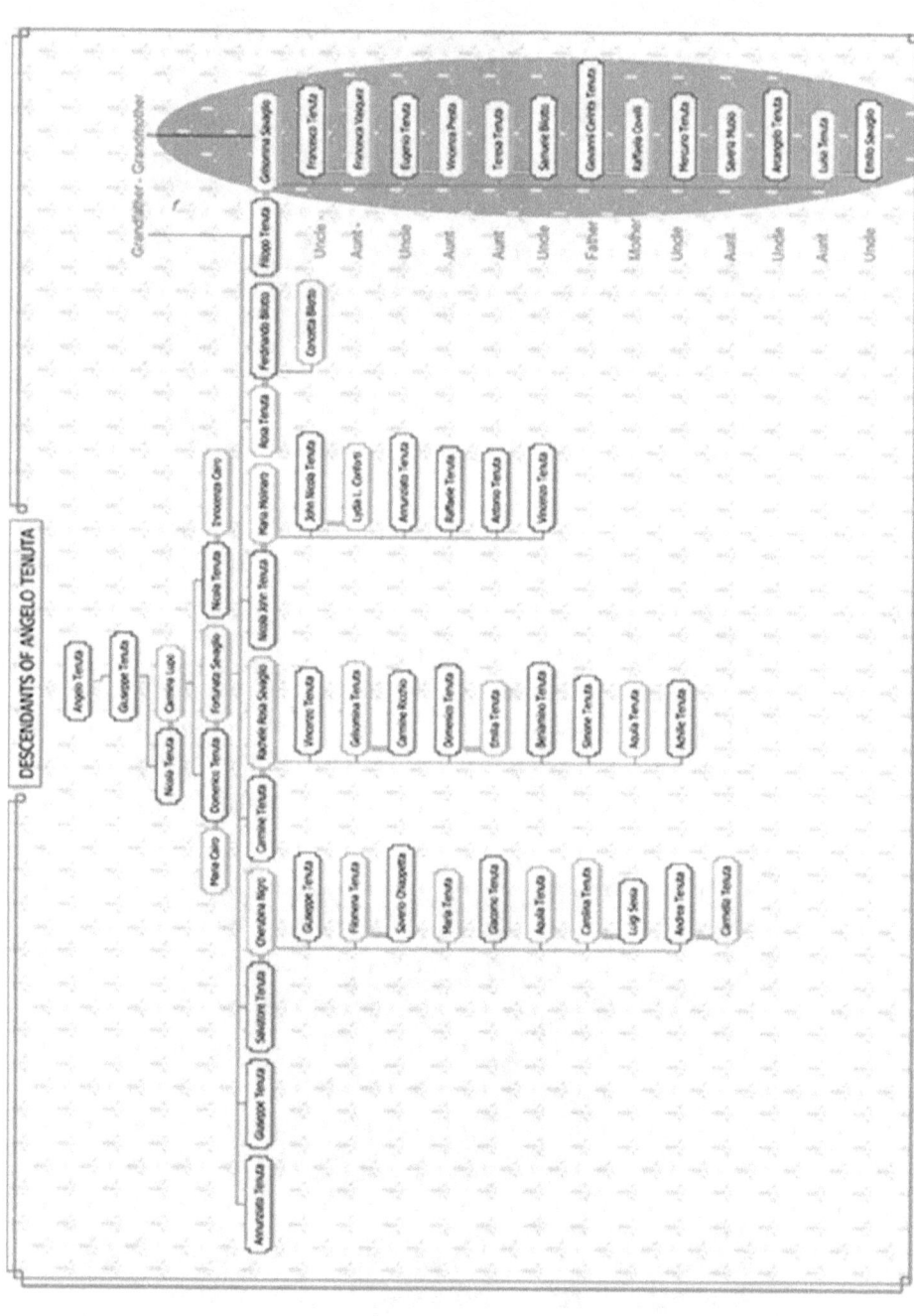

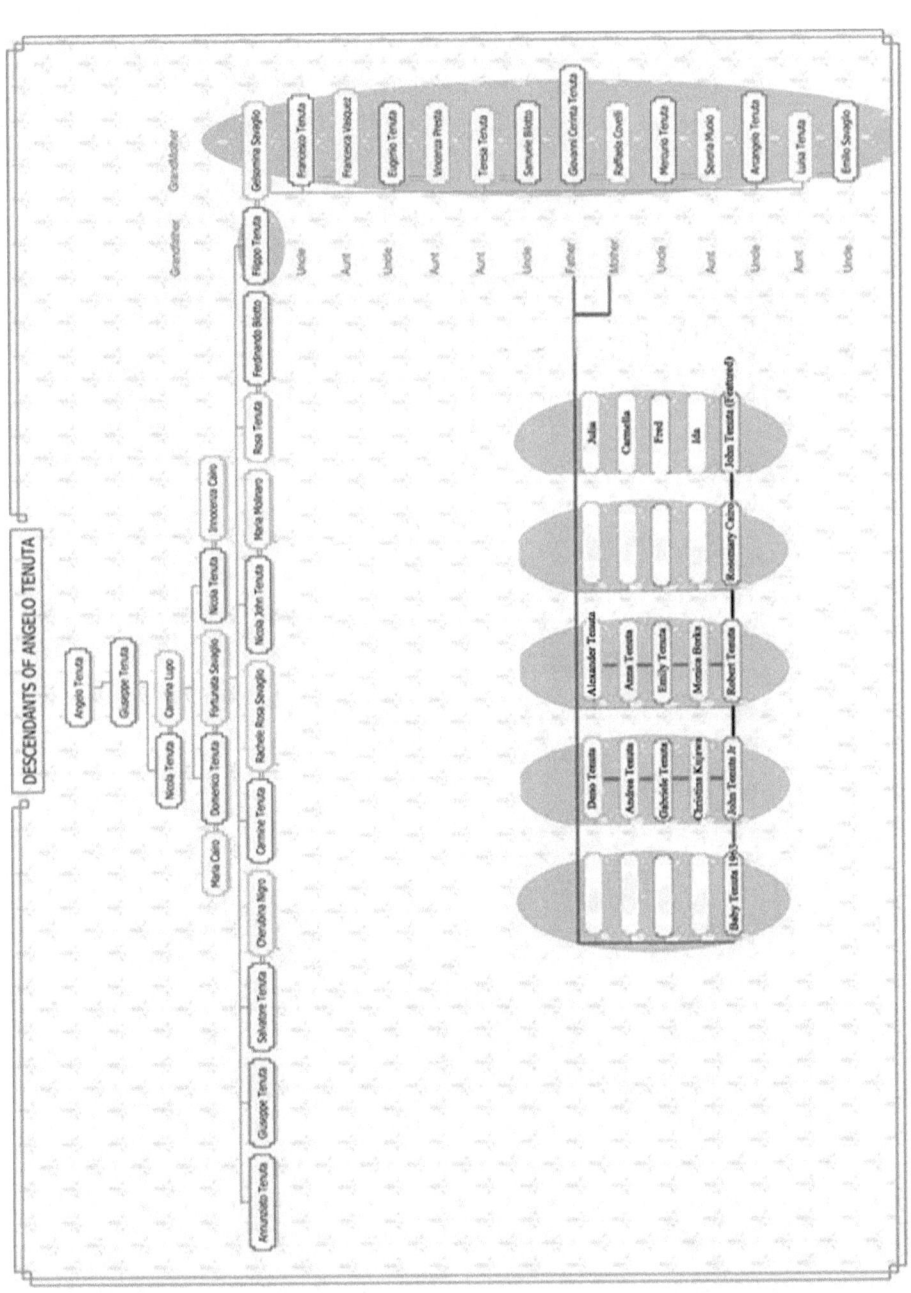

DESCENDANTS OF ANGELO TENUTA

Life of a Barber—DOs & TABOOs, like all great love stories, starts with a journey. This biography portrays a love of family that stretches across the globe, from America to Italy and back, where the Tenuta family values put John Tenuta on a path to love, family, prosperity and liberty.

Born in the United States, immigrated to Italy at the age of three, John survived the ravages World War II. He was raised in the Tenuta Neighborhood outside of the Provence of Cosenza, Italy.

Having first-hand experience of American bombing raids, he tells his story orally due to the fact that his childhood didn't afford him the privilege of an education.

Illiterate and impoverished—from the worst imaginable living conditions of poverty and war—at 18, John returned to the United States and became a successful business owner, homeowner and a loving husband and father in seven years. His family values, integrity and belief in American freedoms motivated him to produce this book: *Life of a Barber—The DOs & TABOOs*.

It has been my unique experience working with John Tenuta, a retired barber, who was born at a time and into circumstances which would have stifled many.

Each section describes different stages of John's life and career as a barber. He considers experience as the best teacher and wishes to depart tips of information, *DOs & TABOOs*, to help others learn from his own experiences and help others avoid obstacles wherever possible.

The *DOs & TABOOs* sections at the end of each chapter are devoted to Johns' thoughts concerning business ethics and family values. Useful or not, they are free advice to anyone who reads *Life of a Barber—The DOs & TABOOs*

In the final chapter, John takes his *DOs & TABOOs* to a more personal family and friend's level. You will read his proscribed strings at several points to stress the importance of his family values.

Definitions for the purpose of this book:

DO—*An action or thought proscribed by society as proper or acceptable to execute*

TABOO—*An action or thought proscribed by society as improper or unacceptable* (Dictionary.com)

John's life, working over barber chairs is full of stories about men who came into his barber shop to get haircuts, talk about their lives, complain about their jobs—and tell barber jokes.

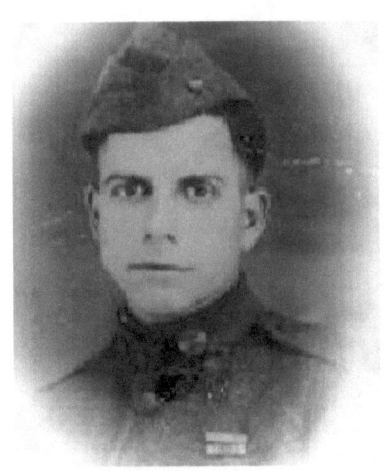

The history of John Tenuta's life begins with his heroic father, World War I veteran Giovanni Tenuta. The Tenuta family has hailed its surname and its ancestry exclusively from Marano Principato for over 200 years.

The veteran Giovanni was born in Marano Principato in 1887. The earliest known picture is this US Army service photo taken in 1919. Giovanni's great-great grandfather, Domenico Tenuta was the first ancestor born in the village in 1807. The village was fittingly named the Tenuta Neighborhood.

Giovanni and his wife Raffaela had five children: Julia, Carmella, Fred, Ida, and John—the principle of our book. John was the last born child in the Tenuta family.

CHAPTER ONE

My Early Years Moving From America To Italy

As far as I can remember, nothing was ever told. No stories were written—that I can say were handed down over the generations about the long history of the Tenuta Family. I would like to tell the story about what went on; what was done, and how I lived from day one—the day I was born—until today.

I was born in Kenosha, Wisconsin in 1934. My father brought our family to Southern Italy when I was three years old. In 1937, we moved to a village named after the generations of the Tenuta family. The Tenuta Neighborhood was in the town of Marano Principato, which is near the province of Cosenza, the capital city of the Calabria region in Southern Italy.

Soon after we moved there, World War II started. We had tough times in our Italian homeland. The Tenuta neighborhood was a small area, about 200 families, surrounded by similar neighborhoods named after the families in those areas. Those villages were called Savaglio, and Ruffolo, and the Covelli neighborhoods, all of which were about one-half mile apart, in different directions. When I was very young, my older sister Ida married a man named Cesare (pronounced "Ceasar") from the Ruffolo neighborhood. Later in my story, I will explain how these family names affected my life in America.

The Tenuta neighborhood was on the side of mountains riddled with tunnels, and there were very few flat areas in the village. Dirt roads would go up or down, but there were very few roads that ran along flat areas. The sky was usually sunny.

One thing I want to tell you—let me put it to you this way: "In Italy, we didn't have very many luxuries. There was no running water. There were no modern toilets, and there was no modern heat. And, why my parents wanted to go back to their homeland of Italy; knowing we didn't have anything with the exception of a little old house and great weather for my mother's health, I don't know. Still, at my age, I wonder why and I don't know why we went back." We stayed in that little old house that my father bought when he was a young man.

My father served and fought in the American military during World War I—the U.S. Army. After moving to back to Italy, he learned that he was eligible for a pension for his military service. He was told to go to the American consulate in Italy to file papers and he would receive a military pension. When my father received his pension, he got about 60 dollars (American) per month to care for our whole family. It was with his pension he was able to provide our family with food, with clothing and pay our electric bills.

In 1938, my brother, Fred, and my sister-Carmela, who were both born in Italy, wanted to go back to United States. So, my father took them back from Italy to Kenosha, Wisconsin to the city I was born. After taking them back to America, my father started his return-journey back home to Italy to live with my mother, my sister and me. I was very young, and my sister Ida was a little older than me.

During his trip back from Kenosha, he arrived in New York to begin his return-journey to Italy, but the owners of the ship he was boarding wouldn't let him on the ship out of the country with his American passport because World War II had started. In order to come back to Italy, he had to return to Kenosha. There, he renounced his American citizenship. He got an Italian passport so he could return to our home in Italy. He held my American birth certificate in a safe place in case I wanted to someday return to the United States.

Once he got his passport to Italy, he boarded a ship in April of 1939 for an over-seas voyage to Europe. He landed in England ten days later. Then he started a long journey across Europe to get back home to us. Getting across Europe during the war meant he had to walk very long distances. He hitched rides on the back of wagons, on fishing boats, and whatever form of transportation he could get. He finally made it back to our home in the Tenuta neighborhood in November—about seven months later.

After my father returned from the United States, our family made arrangements with land owners deep in the Calabria region hillsides to plant vegetable gardens for our food. Sometimes we walked five miles deep into the hills carrying our gardening tools to work the land and tend to our crops. My father and I would dig the soil for planting, and later we would dig the weeds out of the rows. At harvest time, we had to share our harvest with the land owners (usually a 50/50 percent split).

Our neighborhood was more fortunate than other Italian neighborhoods which had no luxuries at all. We at least had small wooden out-houses with benches inside that had holes cut in for toilet seats. There was no toilet paper. For that, people just used wrinkled up newspaper or magazine paper, and sometimes even corn-husks. When you were walking down the street, you had to watch your step. Because when people had to "go," they sometimes just did it on the roads. When women had to relieve themselves, they would just do so discretely in a standing up position trying not to be noticed. There was no disgrace in this, because the conditions were so harsh and poor. In the whole area, there was only one doctor, one priest and one teacher. The town barber was also the dentist, shoemaker and veterinarian.

In the fifteen years I was there, I never had a real bath or a real shower. For water, we hauled small containers from the river to our home for cooking and cleaning, and we washed up from the water we had left over. Sometimes, I saw women bathing in the river. They would wade out into the river as out-of-sight as they could get and lift their dresses up as they entered the water. That way they could bathe themselves. Many women had burn scars around their ankles from standing too close to fireplaces—trying to stay warm in the winter.

Food, clothing and electric were the only necessities we could afford. During my childhood, I usually had one or two pair of trousers, two pair of socks, two shirts, one warm sweater or jacket and a pair of shoes made of canvas. Those were the only cloths I owned, and I was glad to have what clothing I had. When my canvas shoes got wet, they would shrink onto my feet, and sometimes it would take three people to help me pull them off. My socks were made from spun wool from sheep in the area. Their normal color was a woolen cream color, but often my mother would dye the socks to hide the aged and dirty look—usually caused by the fact that my stockings had to last for such a long time. When I got hole in them, my mother repaired them by stitching them back together.

For food, all the families in our village would make bread once per month. There was only one oven in the entire Tenuta neighborhood. Each family had to wait its turn. The bread was usually cornbread. In the summer-time, we had vegetables from our garden such as onions, cucumbers, olives and tomatoes to make salads—the tomatoes were so sweet.

There were times that food was so scarce that we would look through our kitchen area just to find a little bread. When we did find a little bread without mold, we had bread with our salad—and that was our supper. Sometimes, when fruit was in season, we ate fruit. We lived off the fruit trees in the area—sometimes figs, pears, peaches and sometimes apples. Most of the time, the apples we picked were from very high up in the trees. They were usually soft and mushy. To this day, whenever I buy apples, I set them out on the counter to ripen and get mushy, because I enjoy eating apples like the apples I grew up on.

We raised a few chickens to get our eggs. Some of the eggs would hatch into small chicks. Most of those chicks, we would give to the neighbors. But as for meat; we didn't have meat for ages. Once per year, we would have to walk a few miles to a farm near the City of Cosenza to buy a baby pig. We raised it until it was large enough to butcher. We often carried the baby pigs which were usually about two or three weeks old all the way home. Sometimes the baby pigs were large enough that we could lead them with a rope to our home. We would raise them for about ten months, and then we butchered them. The neighbors all joined together during butchering day to make sausage, salami and lard.

On special holidays, my father would buy a piece of lamb for a holiday meal.

When grain was available, the best flour was used to make bread to feed the soldiers first. Then, some people would use the wheat that was left over—the kind of grain that was usually used to feed the pigs to make an awful-tasting white bread.

At six years old, I started going to school. Once per week, on Saturday, I would go to Catechism classes. There was only one teacher in our village. The teacher was very strict. She would punish us kids by striking us with a long round stick across our cold hands. When that happened to me, my hands went numb. Sometimes it took a couple of hours to get movement back in my hands. The rest of the week, I went to school for one-half day, and then I had to go home and stay inside. I lived like a prisoner in my own home, because we never knew if or when the bombing raids were coming. I always wanted to get out of the house in the very worst way.

One day during class, at about the age of six, I had my first experience with a bombing raid near our neighborhood. From then on, the bombings came unexpectedly—we never knew when to expect them. Often there were no warnings or sirens. I remember them being American bombings, because German soldiers were close to our neighborhood; and at certain times, other homes nearby would get bombed causing (collateral) damage—mostly in or near the city of Cosenza about six miles from our home. The bombing raids went on for nearly 4-1/2 years from 1941-42 to 1946.

Our chances for survival were much better if we ran for shelter in the nearby tunnels. So, there were times when we ran from our homes to the tunnels. In the tunnels there were sometimes thirty people at a time—depending on the size of the tunnel or the part of town we were in. The bombs never actually hit our neighborhood, but we ran to the tunnels because we never knew where the bombs were going to land.

When Germans were gunning toward the American planes, shells from their large guns would land in our neighborhood. Once, a shell hit the cement casing next to our window. We came to expect dangerous things like that happening. When the war planes were gone, and the bombing stopped, we all returned to our homes. I thank God we never got hurt.

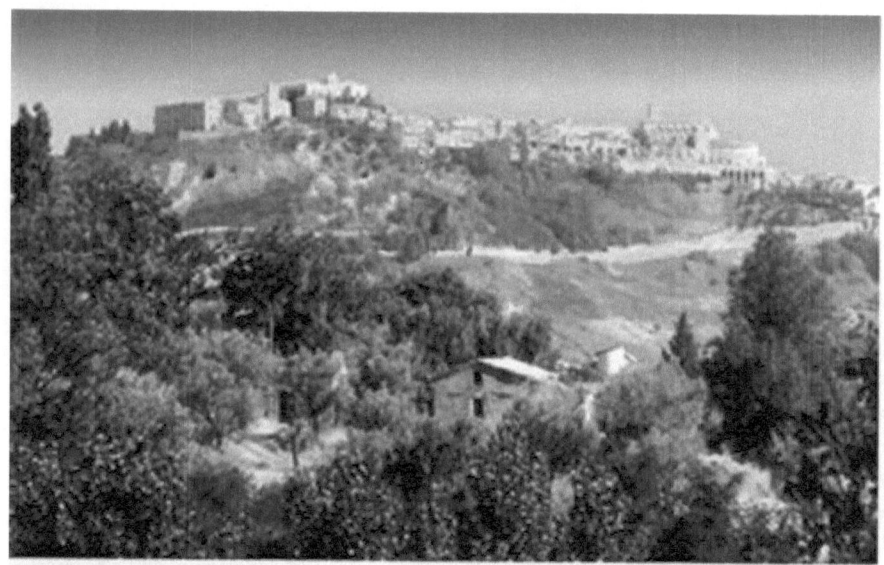

Photo by Al Yeagar

Tenuta Family Farmland - Rende on Hillside Background

Looking closely at the above photo, you can see a couple tunnels in the left side of the hillsides.

World War II finally ended, and we all had to start over rebuilding our homes and our neighborhoods. The homes in our area were not destroyed from bombs, but during the war, nothing was ever done for the up-keep of our homes. The whole area had severely declined. We all started working to make them look nicer by doing repairs that had been avoided during the war. It was our way of surviving the terrible war we had gone through.

In the Tenuta neighborhood, we all started over with the only luxuries we had. Our neighborhood had electricity and one brick-and-stone-built oven that the whole village shared. Most nearby neighborhoods had no luxuries at all.

To get out of the house, I decided to go to the neighborhood barber shop to sweep the floor. Once in a great while, I got a penny for sweeping the floor. The barber shop had one wooden barber's chair and one waiting chair. Most of the boys who hung out in the neighborhood had long hair because there was no extra money for haircuts. As I was sweeping the barber shop floors, I watched the barbers cutting hair, and at age 12, I started giving other neighborhood boys haircuts, I ended up giving most of the neighborhood boys haircuts, and sometimes I even gave the older gentlemen haircuts too. God help them—the way they looked. Nobody had any money—not even a couple of pennies it would have cost them. So, the neighborhood guys came to me. No matter what kind haircut I gave them, or how it looked, they accepted them because it was all they could get. I cut hair in the Tenuta neighborhood until I was 18 years old. For the first couple of years, I cut hair inside my own home or in the homes of other boys or men in the neighborhood.

As mentioned, the town barber was also the town dentist and veterinarian. Once, my father took me to the barber to get my tooth pulled. And, when I saw the barber using the same pair of pliers he had used on a horse's mouth the previous day, I left that place and waited until my father could take me to the city to a real dental office and take care of my tooth.

Starting out in the barber business was a daily challenge. Using the old-fashioned cutting tools presented problems that barbers don't experience using today's modern sheers and automatic clippers.

One day a neighbor asked me to give him a shave. While I was foaming him up, he mentioned he had a problem getting a close shave around his cheek. I told him: "I have just the thing." I took a small wooden ball from a nearby drawer and said: "Just place the ball between your cheek and gum."

He placed it in his mouth and I proceeded to give the man the closest shave he ever experienced. After a few strokes, he asked me in a garbled speech: "And, What if I swallow it?"

"No problem" I said, "Just bring it back tomorrow—like everyone else does." (Anonymous)

When the war was over, my brother Fred suggested that I go into the city of Cosenza to learn the barber business in a professional shop.

So, for the next 2-1/2 years, I traveled each working day into the city to learn by working in professional barber shops. I had to walk 5-1/2 miles to work. My father preferred that I not walk home at night after work, so he gave me money for the return-ride home on the bus.

So, let me tell you what I would do. A few times, I got on the bus and sat near the middle or close to the back. When the conductor came to collect money or punch the passenger tickets, when he reached the middle section, I would sneak past behind him and go sit in the front of the bus—that way I wouldn't have to pay. Once in a while he would pass by me and point his finger at me to let me know he knew I had tricked him. But he was a nice man. And, I rode with him on the bus five days per week. He never gave me hell or hollered at me, and he didn't make me pay. Even though I was only a teenager (15 to 17-years-old), when I got off the bus, I would touch him on the arm and say: "Thank You and Good Night." I picture him today with a big smile on his face, knowing what I (we) had done. He saw me as a respectable and hard-working kid. In those days it was 10-to-15 cents for the bus trip. The following day, when I got back to the city, I would buy myself a piece of candy or fruit with the money I had saved from not having to pay the bus fare.

In 1949, my brother, Fred, returned from America to visit us in Italy. He suggested I come back to The United States and start a life as a barber. He said I could become a successful barber even without an education. I liked what I was doing—cutting hair, so in 1952, at 18 years old, I set out for America to start a career as a barber. Staying in Italy meant I would have had to join the Italian Army. So, it was an easy decision.

In July, my father and I went to Naples to set up my trip for the next month. On August 12, I left home for my trip to America. On the August 13, we arrived in Naples to get my passport stamped. Then on August 14, I started hanging around with my friend Eugene until our religious holiday was over. On Friday, August 15, (called Grey Friday) everything was closed, including the docks, because of the Italian holiday commemorating Santa Madonna dell'Assunta.

Italy is a country of feasts and festivals and Calabria was no exception. Within a 100 km. radius of anywhere in Calabria you can attend a party every day. Many festivals become a part of the local culture. There are people celebrating patron saints, such as, Santa Madonna dell' Assunta. In nearly every town, and village, there are parties and every business gets shut down for the holiday. Today, the holiday is also known as: "Mezzo Augusto." Mezzo Augusto, the August 15th holiday, Assumption Day (like America's Labor Day) is when all Italy, or so it seems, stops work to celebrate.

What Italians are actually celebrating on that day is actually quite interesting because the festival has elements of both the ancient and Christian worlds. First proclaimed by the Emperor Augustus in 18 BC the "Feriae Augusti" originally lasted for all or most of August. It was a time when everyone felt they could relax after the hard work of the harvest and, unusually, a period when the nobility mixed with the laboring classes. The Romans feted the gods of agriculture and those associated with the change of seasons. Roman women feted Diana—The Goddess of Hunting—but also because of her association with the phases of the moon and of maternity.

The festival evolved from being a month-long event to an event celebrated in the second half of August and later became a one-day celebration. Yet in some parts of Italy there are echoes of the ancient, longer feast in the habit of not reopening shops on August evenings. Later on, Christians began to celebrate the Assumption of the Virgin Mary on 15th August and so we have the Mezzo Augusto of today.

During the day, you could hear a pin drop in the center of many Italian towns as people gathered in the countryside or in their houses with relatives and friends to celebrate. But the night is a different matter in many towns and even a small village may hold a fireworks display. (Wikipedia)

On August 16, 1952, I boarded the ship to America. I never saw my parents again. It seems like it was yesterday. I was sea-sick the whole voyage. There were a couple of nice ladies on the ship who came to look in on me, to make sure I was OK, during the whole voyage.

On the voyage to America, there was a famous and accomplished Irish-style singer, Frank Parker, who was entertaining the guests. When his entertaining was finished, he circulated from table to table and talked to the guests and shook our hands. Parker is remembered for the honor of being part of classic television, making regular performances on the famed show *Arthur Godfrey and His Friends* from 1950 to 1956. Arthur Godfrey's straightforward, informal style—along with his tendency to poke fun at his sponsors—made him one of the most popular radio personalities of the time. Parker also appeared as panelist on *TV's Masquerade Party.*

We could have made it into New York in nine days, but the Sunday before our arrival, the ship started slowing down. The New York harbor was backed up and there was no place to dock. It took an extra day to dock the ship.

We finally arrived in New York on Monday morning at 9:00 am.

DOs & TABOOs

DO*: It is great to have barber who can cut your hair and repair your shoes in the same shop.*

TABOO*: It is not so good to pick a barber who is also the town-dentist and veterinarian—especially if he is willing to pull a bad-tooth with the same pair of pliers that he used pulling a tooth from a horse's mouth the previous day.*

DO*: The tradition of making homemade bread has been around my whole life, and eating bread with salads is one of my favorite meals.*

TABOO*: Making bread from left-over grains you get an awful-tasting white bread, but even worse tasting in my opinion is "Wonder Bread."*

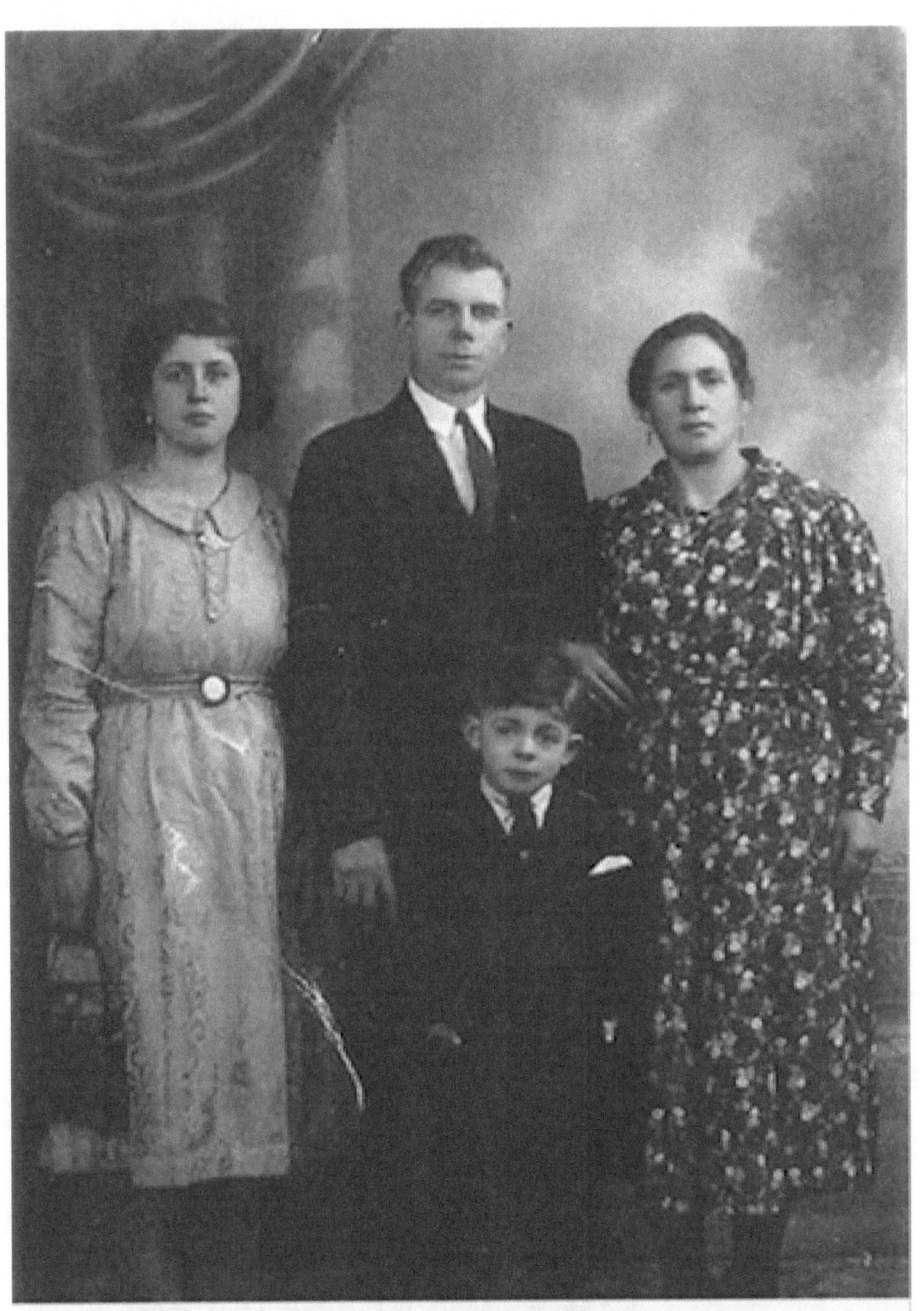

From Left to Right: John's sister Ida, his father Giovanni,
his nephew Aldueno and his mother Raffeala

CHAPTER TWO

Landing In America And Starting My Career

I finally got off the ship in New York. Seeing New York was the best experience in my life. The most gorgeous site was the Statue of Liberty. In those days, the Statue of Liberty represented the world-wide symbol of the liberty of life. I realized I was finally in the place where a person could do anything they want. I knew I was in a land where I could become a rich person—even without an education. Nobody in the United States ever told me I had to go to school to find a job. But I knew I had to go to work to pay for my room and board.

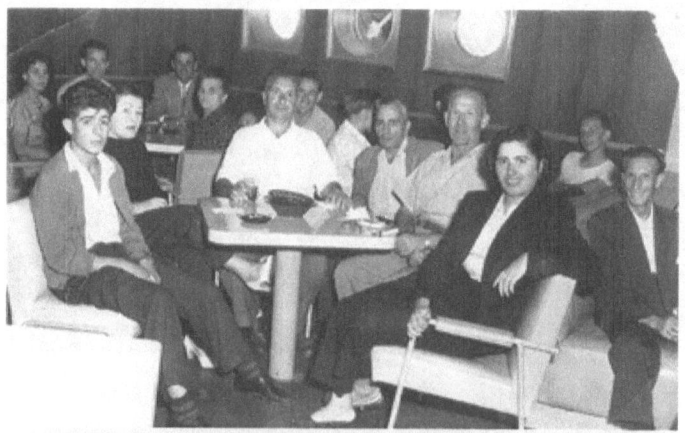

From Left: John Tenuta at 18, lady traveler, gentleman (1) from California, man traveler, gentleman (2) from Chicago and at rigth, one of the nice ladies who looked in on John during his sea-sick voyage.
Genitlemen (1 & 2) continued on with John to Chicago.

Three of us men got off the ship together. There was one gentleman from Chicago, one from California and me. The two men knew their way around New York and helped me make it to the train to Chicago. The first thing the three of us did, when we got off the ship, was go to a grocery store and bought some lunch meat and a loaf of American-style bread—Wonder Bread—to take with us on the train ride. At 6 pm, we got on the train. We arrived in Chicago the following morning at 8 am. My two sisters, Carmela and Julia and Julia's husband Ralph were there waiting for me.

I lived with Carmela and my brother-in-law, Tony, for about one year. But I didn't get along Tony because he was—well, just say: "One-of-a-Kind"—just to let people know what a no-good person he was to Carmella. I didn't like the way he treated her, calling her names—like: "Stupid" and other awful names I would not want to repeat. He often said mean things to her if she didn't do things his way. Eventually, Tony started treating me in the same mean way. One day he suggested that I move out. So, I moved out and stayed at the YMCA. I ended up living at the "Y" for nearly five years. Carmela only stayed with Tony because she was from the old school—when women didn't leave their husbands.

Tony had four sisters who were very much like him. The way Tony and his sisters acted toward their spouses seemed like a way of life for them. I never saw those people have a good sense of humor. The times I saw them, they were always mean to their spouses. Maybe in their own way they loved each other, but they didn't show it. To each other, they always acted sarcastic. To others, they acted like nice people.

During my childhood, I always planned to someday move back to Kenosha, Wisconsin, so while I was in Chicago looking for work and making career decisions, I went to Kenosha for a visit. When I returned to Chicago, a friend of mine, Alex Vercillo, told me he knew a barber named Joe Perelli, who was looking for another barber for his shop. I met Perelli and he suggested that I work with him and said he would help me get into the barber business. So I stayed in Chicago and worked with him.

Working in the barber business in Chicago was much different than the conditions I was familiar. Back in Italy, I didn't even have a pair of automatic hand-clippers. Perelli offered to send me to the barber college for a few days to learn how to use the automatic hand-clippers and put the towels and hair-cutting gowns around the customers' necks the professional way. Learning at the barber college was free for a short time, so I took him up on his offer.

Before working with Perelli, I just wore normal shirts—whatever I had. He told me that I had to wear a nice shirt and a tie at work. Since then, I have always worn a nice shirt and tie and a nice barber coat while working. Dressing like a professional barber was a good lesson that I continued throughout my whole career.

A week later, I started working at *"Joe Perelli's Barber Shop."* Perelli was a nice old-timer. He treated me well—like his "Main Man." He always took my advice in things that were important in business matters. In return, I worked at the barber shop and treated the business like it was my own. I worked with Perelli until 1960.

One day a young man came into the barber shop and said: "I want my hair cut just like The Beatles."

So I told him: "Ok, No problem."

The young man sat down and fell asleep.

When he woke up he saw I had shaved his head completely bald.

The young man became startled when he saw his bald head and said: "Hey, The Beatles don't look like this."

I smiled and answered: "They would if they came here!" (Anonymous)

I could have been paid like barber businesses pay today—by the haircut. Perelli had confidence in me, and he paid me a good salary. Being paid by salary was considered very respectable in those days. It gave me a sense of stability and respectability.

The shop was an easy-going place to work. Our rent was cheap and the electric was only six or seven dollars per month. Our gas bill for heating was 10 to 12 dollars during the colder winter months. We paid our bills just down the block at the currency exchange. The only other bill we had to be concerned with was the rent which we usually paid in cash.

Apart from haircuts, the only other responsibility I had to concern myself with was keeping the shop clean, which included cleaning the windows. We had a showcase full of hair tonic that we sold for 50 to 75 cents per bottle.

In Chicago, I hung out with friends who worked together in a Wonder Bread factory. For extra money, I worked with them part-time during the night-shift at the factory—from 6 pm until 2 am. I usually got about 5-1/2 to six hours of sleep, and then I got up and went back to work at the barber shop. There, I worked from 9 am until 5 pm. So, between jobs, I didn't get much sleep.

The Chevrolet Impala came out in 1958. It was the most popular car on the market that year. The Impala signified the rompin' and stompin' pride of the American highways that only top-ended at 100 mph, but its thundering V-8 engine was capable of burning long black rubber stripes on the pavement from a dead stop. I bought a black one, knowing General Motors' Body by Fisher™ only painted perfect-fitting auto bodies black because the nature of black paint is that it shows every imperfection. Whenever a person bought a black car, it was considered the best fitting and highest quality auto body manufacturers could produce.

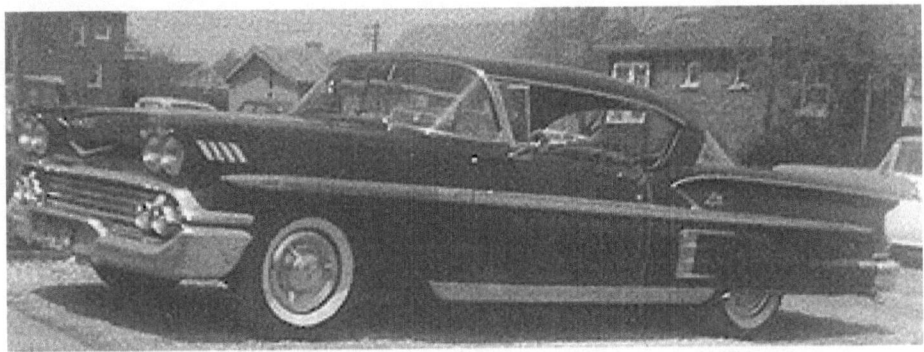

The area of Chicago where I lived and worked was a close Italian neighborhood and most of the people knew each other.

I worked for Perelli for about seven or eight years. During that time I drove to the hospital to shave men a couple of times per week. The price for a haircut was 75 cents, and the price for a shave was one dollar. One day, a gentleman named Fred Cairo came into the barber shop. He told me he had a brother in the hospital that needed a shave, so I drove to the hospital twice per week to shave his brother Frank.

One Saturday night, after work, I stopped by the hospital to give Frank a shave. His wife, Adeline, was with him. It was the first time I met her, and I noticed right away that the Cairos had a special quality about their relationship. I couldn't help but notice how Frank and Adeline always spoke to each other with a smile. It was a quality that I saw a very rare. At that time, I didn't know that they would eventually become my father—and mother-in-laws in years to come. I think Frank had four or five brothers and two sisters. Frank was born in Italy. His mother brought him to America. Adeline was born in the United States. The Cairo family and I developed a decent friendship.

One day, while I was shaving Frank, his daughter Rosemary came in from the hallway. My first thought was: "She was the most precious thing I had ever seen." On first sight, I knew I could like her very much. I had dated other girls before that, but when I saw her, I just knew that she could be *The One*. The whole time I was giving Frank a shave, one of my eyes was on the father, and the other eye was on the daughter.

By coincidence, a few months later, Perelli asked me to drive him to the Cairo's home. It was then that I got to know Rosemary a little more. "I checked her out." Again, I remember thinking that she was exactly the kind of beautiful person I was always hoping for (as a wife).

A few weeks later, on a Sunday afternoon, Perelli asked me to give him another ride to the Cairo's home. It was then I got the courage to ask Rosemary: "Could you give me your phone number?" A couple minutes later, she gave me the piece of paper (with her number).

The first time we dated was in 1956—right before Christmas. I remember the first movie we went to see. It was musical named *Pal Joey* with Frank Sinatra, Kim Novak and Rita Hayworth. We dated for a couple of years.

Saturday nights we went out on dates—usually to the movies. We spent most of our Sundays with her parents. The four of us would spend whole days together playing Italian card games with names such as "Briscola" and "Scupa." Her parents liked it that we spent time with them. They weren't so much watching Rosemary as much as they were watching that she was in good hands.

Rosemary also had a bunch of cousins. Two of them, Rose and Pat, were very close to her. We hung out with them then, and we were close to them for the rest of Rosemary's life. They were like Rosemary's sisters.

Our first Christmas together, I wanted to buy Rosemary a special present. I bought her a light blue sweater. When she saw it, she told me it was the most special gift she had ever gotten from anybody.

For her birthday, in 1957, I bought tickets for a theater play house performance. That night would turn out to be one of the greatest nights of my life. I also made plans to have dinner at Jonny's Steak House in downtown Chicago. But, when we got to the theater play house, she looked at the billboard, and I could tell by the look on her face, the play wasn't something she really wanted to see. Instead, she wanted to go to the movie theater to see the musical: *South Pacific* starring Rossano Brazzi and Mitzi Gayner.

Well—Rosemary was the love of my life. It was her birthday, and I would do anything to please her. We knew the movie theater was only about one-half mile away, so we decided to walk the streets to see the movie and have dinner afterwards—even though the temperature was 10 degrees below zero.

Snow falling and it was cold. We were dressed classy. I wore a cashmere topcoat over my suit with Floor-Shined™ shoes. Rosemary was dressed to the "Nines" with high heels. The whole time we walked, she held my arm. We talked and laughed and avoided slipping on the icy sidewalks.

After the movie, we walked another half mile back toward Jonny's Steak House for dinner and then back to my car. Then, it started snowing real heavy. Soon there were 12 more inches of snow on the ground. It became difficult getting her back home. I had my new Chevy Impala, but I didn't have snow tires or chains, because in those days they were rarely used. Her home was on one of the side-streets, and it took four attempts from different side streets to finally make it onto her street to get her home. We final arrived at her home very late—after 12:30 am. When I finally pulled into her parent's driveway, I made about half way into the drive and stopped the car.

That night and the next night, I stayed on a sofa in the Cairo's home until the roads were clear and safe enough to drive.

I knew by that time I wanted Rosemary in my life forever.

I was driving her home after one of our next dates when I came up with the courage to ask her the *BIG* question. I looked over at her and asked: "What is the chance that I could have you in my life?" She was quite. Then, I looked at her again and asked: "Do I have a chance to have you in my life—*forever?*"

When we arrived in her driveway, I finished my cigarette and we sat in the car for a short time. Right before she went in, I said: "If I had marriage in mind, you didn't give me an answer." I asked her if I had hope or a chance. I told her that I didn't want to lose her.

She looked at me and asked: "What comes first?"

I answered with one word: *"LOVE."*

She looked at me and smiled. I told her: "From day one, I fell in love with you."

I took her in the house, kissed her, and I went home.

I called her about 9:30 the next morning. When she answered the phone, she told me that she didn't sleep for half of the night. When I heard the sound of her voice, my heart felt like it stopped. She said:

"The reason I didn't sleep was because; I felt I should have told you last night that I love you too. And I don't want to l lose you either."

I knew, finally, I would have someone to call my own.

The following night, we were parked in the same place in her parent's old driveway. Rosemary asked me if I would talk to her parents about the idea of us getting married. She asked me to ask them in a proper and traditional way. I told her yes, and I asked them.

Frank and Adeline both agreed it was a good decision for us to get married. When the subject about paying for the wedding came up, Adeline pointed her finger at the old man, and the father offered to pay for the wedding. There was something charming about the high hopes they had for Rosemary.

Soon after, we started looking at wedding rings. After looking, Rosemary said she found the kind of ring she liked. It was called an emerald-cut diamond. I wrote the name down on a piece of paper, in broken English, and put it in my wallet. The next day, I went to a Jewish Jeweler and found a one-karat diamond with a quarter-karat diamond on each side—emerald cut. I knew she wore a size seven. I bought it. In July, I put the ring on her finger, and Frank took us all out to celebrate.

One evening, I was going out with Rosemary. It was at a time when I was getting in real close with Rosemary's family. Her mother Adeline asked me to take off my shirt. I was a little embarrassed at the time. It seemed like a big sin to take my shirt off in front of my girlfriend's mother, but the reason she wanted me to remove my shirt was so she could measure it and fashion me some real nice barber coats. Barbers used to wear the old-style cotton jackets which were just above the knee.

She made me some really nice professional looking barber coats with mid-length sleeves and square bottoms—much like the ones you see the doctors wear today. She must have made me 20 to 25 of those barber coats over the years. They were the "Real Thing"—nice enough that when it was 100 degrees, I didn't feel the heat. She made them with a nice zipper that zipped up the front just high enough to see the fancy shirts and ties that went along with my ensemble. I think that was Adeline's way of welcoming me to the family.

We planned for at least a one-year engagement. While making plans, we also talked about where we would like to live after we got married. Early on, Frank and Adeline suggested that we live with them. But in 1959, about January or February, Rosemary and I decided to look for apartments.

I stayed at the "Y" quite a while after I proposed to Rosemary. I eventually moved into our apartment before we got married, but we didn't go there together much. Whenever we went to my apartment, it was just for a short time—to pick something up—but we never stayed long. It was extremely important for me to show her and her parents that kind of respect. Saving intimate love making for after our marriage was the most cherished wedding gift we could possibly give to each other. Everything and every day from that day forward was an extension of the love we created on that day.

With the new apartment, my expenses went up from 60 to 80 dollars per month, which included utilities. The only other expenses I had were for my car and a phone. Once I got the apartment, we started making serious plans for our wedding.

We decided to hold the wedding at Saint Daniel's Catholic Church and hold the reception at Jaycees Restaurant.

DOs & TABOOs

DO: *It's ok to make plans where you want to live way before you get married.*

TABOO: *In those days, it was not ok take advantage of your bachelor apartment before you get married. After all, what's left if you experience all the intimacy and leave nothing for after marriage?*

CHAPTER THREE

Marrying Rosemary And Starting A Life Together

Rosemary and I were married on June 13, 1959. There were about 200 people at our wedding. We went to Fort Lauderdale for 11 days on our honeymoon. Where ever we went, we dressed nice. One evening, a guy came over to our dinner-table and offered to take our picture for two dollars. That's the picture I carry in my wallet today.

During our honeymoon, we usually stayed inside until about 7 pm, because it was so hot and humid in Florida. Then we would hit the streets. We went to nice restaurants and dancing. I wasn't much of a dancer, but I would tell her: "I'll walk with you."

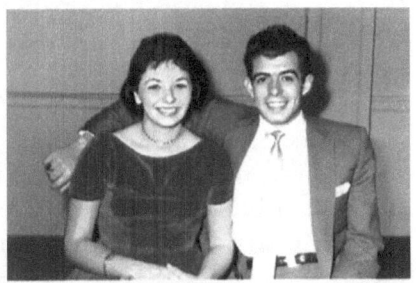

After we got back from our honeymoon, we both went back to work. At the time, Rosemary worked with her father as an office girl. I still worked at *Joe Perelli's Barber Shop*.

In 1960, I left *Joe Perelli's Barber Shop* because many of the people (our clients) were leaving the area. The State of Illinois had bought up much of the land on the west side of the city to build the University of Chicago.

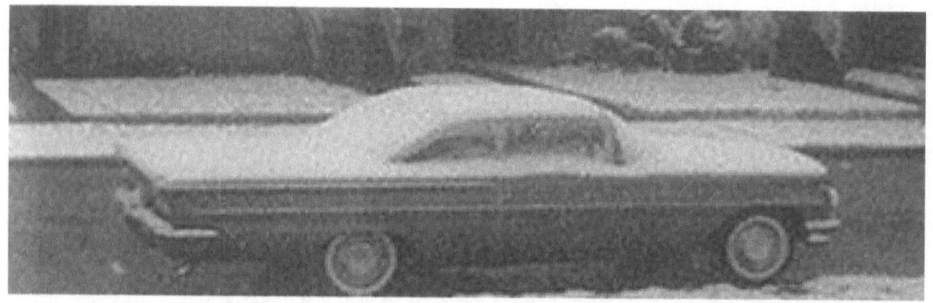

This is the 1960 grey Pontiac I bought after I got married.

I bought my first barber shop a little further West near the City on South Cicero. Originally it was named *Ideal Barber Shop*. I changed the name to *John's Barber Shop*. It had an old fashion barber pole on the outside, and I had neon-light sign made for the front window that read: *John's Barber Shop*. From day one, the only people who worked for me were a second barber and an accountant to take care of my book-keeping. When I started my first shop, the price for a haircut went up to a couple of bucks. The rent at my own barber shop started at 40 dollars per month. My barber shop had four chairs. The barber shop was like a second home for me and the guys. Many of the guys would come into the barber shop and confide in me and tell their stories. Ninety-five percent of the customers who came into my shop were once per week customers.

Rosemary became pregnant in November of 1960. She had our first boy, Robert, in August of 1961. Our first child was a smooth pregnancy. From then on, I had to continue to work to support my family. We bought our first home on LaPorte Avenue around the same time. Everything seemed to happen at once. Along with the marriage and child came a lot of responsibility. But I had Rosemary's help taking care of our home and child. Her effort in the home and her great attitude really helped us make it through.

When Rosemary started working other jobs away from her father, she went to work for the Sears and Roebuck Company. Sears gave us medical benefits. She worked there for 1-1/2 years. At seven months pregnant, Sears gave Rosemary 175 dollars to pay for Robert's delivery, so the hospital and doctor bills only cost us 170 dollars out of our own pocket.

In 1963, Rosemary became pregnant again, but she lost the baby by miscarriage at about 4-1/2 months into her pregnancy. Those days doctors didn't feel it was a good idea to mention things about the babies who didn't make it—even if you knew the baby was a boy or a girl. The doctor told me not to tell Rosemary the baby was a girl. That was really a tough thing to go through all alone.

We waited for another 1-1/2 years, and then we started planning for another baby. Two years later, we had our second son John in 1965. During her pregnancy with John, Rosemary had to take it very easy. When John was born, we had no insurance at all. Between the Doctor's fee of $380.00 and hospital bill, it cost us about 500 dollars. In those days a three-day hospital stay was around 30 to 35 dollars per day.

We always lived within our means. As a rule, if we could not afford things by paying cash for them, we would not buy them.

Things also got a little slow at work because long hair came into fashion. At the time, I already had my children, so I did take on some part-time jobs.

After a couple of years in my own business, my customer, Joe Gross, came into the barber shop and told me to turn on the television. To my surprise, President John F. Kennedy had been shot. It was a shock to hear such a thing could happen here in the United States. When I first heard the news, the President was not yet declared dead, but I watched and waited moment by moment for the news of his fate. I think when his death was announced, that is when people in our country started losing faith in the people running the country and our society. I will never forget the moment CBS News Anchor Walter Cronkite announced the death of the President with tears in his eyes.

I often heard rumors that Vice President, Lynden B. Johnson, would never have been elected as President on his own (merits). Some people suspected that he had the most to gain by the death of President Kennedy. First, a lone gunman, Lee Harvey Oswald, was accused of the shooting.

Before a full investigation could take place, the following Sunday, Oswald was shot by a man named Jack Ruby. There were many rumors that the killing of Oswald, who claimed he was a "Patsy," was part of a cover-up. In the end, Ruby admitted that he alone killed Oswald.

There were many conspiracy theories that came up about the assassination of Kennedy—from naming Lee Harvey Oswald as the lone assassin—to conspiracy theories of multiple shooters. Almost 30 years later, a movie about a conspiracy theory suggesting multiple shooters came out in theaters. Perhaps no one will ever really know what happened. The way the entire situation went down, the investigation ended with no certain way for anyone to ever discover the real truth. That is the sort of thing that causes people to lose faith in our country.

Kennedy supported the space program with the goal of Americans being the first man to land on the moon. Americans later landed on the moon, but he never lived to see it happen.

A few years later, in 1968, his brother Senator Robert F. Kennedy was assassinated. I always felt that someone had it in for the Kennedys. It was rumored that if the third bother Senator Edward M. Kennedy had run for president that he too would have been assassinated. He never ran for president, but he stayed in the Senate his entire life.

Cities were busing students around to different districts to integrate African Americans into our schools.

Four years before we got married, Rosemary went to visit her uncle in New Orleans. She told me a story about an experience she had on a New Orleans bus ride. There were two empty seats in the front of the bus. Two young black women got on the bus and sat down in the empty seats. The bus driver told them to move to the back of the bus. Rosemary did not understand why those young women were treated in such a way. She never judged people like that.

In 1968, Civil Rights Leader Martin Luther King was also assassinated. The American people became more divided.

As we experienced these things, we just tried to move on in our own life.

Friends of mine thought Rosemary and I were loaded with money, but the truth was: In the barber business, I just gave the landlord whatever money I could afford. The monthly payments at the barber shop were very small. And because I stayed with him for so long, the rent rarely went up—just a few bucks here and a few bucks there. When I put a few extra bucks together, I usually put it into the house to pay down the mortgage. My first house payments were 116 dollars per month. At that time, it seemed like big money.

It took us about nine years to pay off the mortgage on our first home. Many times we felt like we cheated ourselves out of luxuries. We could have spent our extra money on luxuries such as vacations, but we chose to be responsible. We worked hard and smart to get ourselves ahead. And we always felt it was important to be money-smart.

Rosemary was a stay-at-home wife and mother. I was the sole bread-winner for fourteen years of our marriage. We always ate healthy. Our family had home-cooking every night. If I ever had a craving for a special dish, it was almost always there waiting for me when I got home from work. Rosemary always took care of me in such ways.

I raised my children at a time when the economy was good. Everybody seemed to be working. We made good friends. Everybody was nice to us. Our friends all respected each other. I also had a good clientele. It seems like I always had a little part-time job. At first, I closed the barber shop on Sundays and Wednesdays. Sundays were always a church day for our family and our friends. From time to time I worked on Wednesdays, because the other barbers were closed and also took Wednesdays off.

About that time, I was getting more active in our church. I thought that I should share my faith with my customers more than I had been doing lately. So the next morning when the sun came up and I got up out of bed and thought: "Today I am going to share my faith with the first man that walks through my barber shop door."

Soon after I opened my shop the first man came in and said, "I want a shave!"

I said: "Sure, just sit in the seat and I'll be with you in a moment."

I went in the back and prayed a quick desperate prayer saying: "God, my first customer just came in and I'm going to share my faith with him. So give me the wisdom to know just the right thing to say to him. Amen."

Then, I quickly came out with my razor knife in one hand and a Bible in the other while saying "Good morning sir. I have a question for you . . . Are you ready to die?" (Anonymous)

The rules barbers in Chicago went by were set by the Barber's Union. The days of the week that barbers worked were even set by the union. Once, the barbers all got together and complained about working—having to work on Wednesdays. Then, there was a vote among union barbers and the work-week changed from having Sundays and Wednesdays off to having Sundays and Mondays off. We didn't buck the system in those days because labor unions were very powerful.

One of the most important things we did in those days was investing to get ahead. Once, Rosemary and I had in our minds to buy a piece of investment property. Later, we bought a small apartment building with six apartments. The investment worked out well for us. I decided to take on a part-time job driving a whiskey truck to earn some extra money after we bought the rental property.

Our investment property was just another example of what a person of my time could do to prosper without an education. Everything I learned, including making investments, I learned from working in the barber shop. I learned about investing by reading the newspapers and magazines and getting tips by talking to people—mostly my customers.

I learned how to communicate well with people. That was the old school. I always kept friendships with my customers. I never denied to customers what I had in mind to do in matters of business or what I had done. They learned to trust me and confide in me. I was well-treated. In return, I treated them well.

During that time, the Catholic Archdioceses from our congregation was calling out for someone in the congregation to administer Holy Communion at Mass. At the time, I wasn't comfortable with the order because I felt a little bit inferior due to my inability to write. The church required Administers of Holy Communion to go to classes—which meant that I had to write. The idea that the congregation would discover I could not write was not something I wanted to experience. I had a hard time getting past my feelings about not writing even though I heard stories and watched one of those television shows, like *60 Minutes*, that once aired a story about the original owner of the Las Vegas Dunes Hotel, who also could not read nor write.

A brief history of the Las Vegas Dunes: The Dunes Hotel was one of the early hotels on the Las Vegas strip, opening its doors in 1955. Together with the Sands and Desert Inn hotels, it was known as one of the Three Kings of Las Vegas. The Dunes was also made famous by recruiting star performers such as Frank Sinatra to sing at the hotel, in an effort to lure the paying golfers into the casinos. Still struggling, though, even with the might of Frank and Company, it opened Las Vegas's first topless show called Minsky's Follies in 1957. (Wikipedia)

Being unable to write was a just a hard thing for me to deal with openly, so for a long time, I didn't administer Holy Communion in our congregation, even though I would have liked to do so. However, now I serve Holy Communion weekly.

Everything in my life was built around my family. Rosemary and I had the best relationship. I think perhaps the way I saw Rosemary's parents, Frank and Adeline, speak to each other with a smile is where I learned to be the same way with Rosemary and, of course, her with me. That was so important.

We never had any arguments. We never had any misunderstandings. If she ever had to tell me something, she would tell me with a smile. She never got excited or told me that I did the wrong thing, or said anything with that kind of negative attitude. Rosemary never had hard feelings for anybody. We never had an argument in 49 years of marriage. Once in a while, I would get excited about something, and she would just come up to me and put a smile on me—a mile long. Rosemary would say: "Don't get excited-relax—Things will work out!" She always had her special way of settling me down.

I never played the ponies. In the beginning of my career as a barber shop owner, there was a guy down the street who would book the horses.

On the top of my hair tonic showcase we had a rubber pad about eight inches round in plain sight. One day, the guy asked me if he could use the rubber pad. He told me that from time to time some guys were going to put small pieces of paper under the pad, and later in the afternoon, he would pick up the pieces of paper. He said that was all that I had to do to make some easy money. Well I asked him: "What's the pay?" He didn't answer right away.

So, a few days later, he came by the barber shop and gave me nine dollars. I asked him what it was all about, and he told me that the people who leave their papers here are playing the ponies, and he told me that he booked the horses. He also told me that the barber who owned the shop before me allowed him to use the barber shop in the same way.

Later in the afternoon, one of my customers came into the barber shop and told me that if I get caught booking the horses, I could go to jail. That's all I had to hear. I couldn't see me going to jail for booking someone else's horses. The next time that guy came in, I said: "No More!" I told him, I didn't want to go to jail, and I explained that I was too young and there wasn't anyone there going to protect me. The bookie told me that he didn't blame me, and we never did that again.

I just allowed that one time and the first nine dollars stayed with me. But I didn't want any part of anything that would put my business at risk. Since then, I have stayed out of those kinds of things that could get me into trouble. I have never done bad things to anybody, and I have never given anybody the cold shoulder. My customers appreciate it.

I was a 29 or 30-year-old business owner. One day, an inspector from the government came into the barber shop—just to look around. He showed me his badge and told me he was checking on the small businesses in the area. He asked to see my books. So, I showed him my records. He asked me if I paid estimated taxes. I told him yes. After he looked at my books, he saw my bottles of hair tonic for sale and asked if I sold them in my barber shop. Again, I said yes.

He looked at the bottles and said: "I don't see any sales tax."

And then I responded to him with a rhetorical question: "Sir, at 75 cents per bottle?"

And then with a second question, I asked: "Sir, When is your birthday?"

He told me his birthday, and after he answered, I explained to him: "Sir, if you come in to get a haircut on your birthday and you tell us it is your birthday, then, we give you a free bottle of hair tonic. It would be pretty hard to compute sales tax on such a give-a-way item."

The inspector started to laugh and said: "I give you a lot of credit as a small business-person." The inspector sat down with me and my other barber to talk for about an hour. We talked like we were friends forever. Once he left, I still felt a little skeptical—thinking he was going to try to find something to do to me, but I never heard from him again—knock on wood! In fifty years, I never had the government come down on me for trying to cheat them on taxes. But I have always paid my taxes, and if the IRS ever called me, I was always ready and would show them my records in black and white. When you are in business, you have to show that you make money. They seem to want to know what you make on the side. So I always kept good records.

I went to work every work day to support my family. I lived for the idea raising them the best way I could. Thank God for the barber business that we never went without necessities.

As a barber, I ran into all kinds of people. I didn't go to school for very long, but as a barber, I learned how to respect people and to get people to respect me.

Early in my career, I started reading in my spare time, and I learned to read pretty well. I have done a lot of things in life—that even if I had gone through ten years of education—I would not have done any better. I learned almost everything about business in my barber shop. Today, I read many things; I read newspapers and magazines, I read things for The Knights of Columbus meetings, because in the time I sit in the barber shop, (when it's not busy), I have to do something—so I read.

Ninety-nine percent of the people who come into the barber shop are nice people. Once in a while, I get a person who is a little bit nasty. Maybe he doesn't know what he wants. Maybe he is just having a bad day. Or, maybe he just doesn't like my attitude. Well, I only have to spend about 15 minutes with him, so I can be patient and put up with him. Once he is gone, I figure: "God Bless Him." If he comes back, I do the best that I can. If he doesn't come back, I lose him, but soon I have someone who will replace him. Talking to those customers respectfully is a job in itself. I enjoy every bit of it. Even today, I don't have to work, because I am 77 years old, but I enjoy being with my customers.

Throughout the years, I supported my family pretty well. For a period of time, I didn't even have any hospitalization insurance. I raised two boys, and I thank God during that time, we never had any major problems that required any of our family going into the hospitals.

I will never forget the one time I borrowed one thousand dollars from Sears & Roebucks Company for a new car. Sears financed the car for 18 months. With interest included, the car cost me 1,370 dollars. The interest on the loan was 370 dollars. At that time, I also had one thousand dollars saved in the bank, but the banks only paid 62 dollars in interest—when I kept our money in a bank savings account. The way banks charged such high interest rates on loans, yet they gave you so little interest payments on a saving accounts didn't seem fair to me. So from that time on, I decided if I didn't have the money to pay for a car with cash, I did not buy a car. Up until today, that's what I have done my whole life—pay cash. From 1960 to 1972, I supported my wife, raised my kids and owned my own business on a cash basis, and I only worked at my barber shop and small part-time jobs. I didn't have to take out loans.

In 1972, we bought a piece of investment property on credit. The property paid for itself by rent paid by tenants. But when I bought the building, I invested everything we had so the mortgage would be a little cheaper. We kept the investment property for almost 18 years. The money we made off the property helped us pay for our new house in Orland Park.

Once, Rosemary's Uncle Fred came into my barber shop for a haircut. He asked how we were doing. I explained to him that I had recently spent every penny I had on the investment property and that long hair had come in and things in the barber business were a getting a little slow. So he suggested I come to work for him part-time on the loading docks where he worked as a foreman. I wanted to have a few extra bucks on hand so I took that second job. He said I could come in whenever I want. He said I could come in at 6 pm and when I thought I had enough, I could just go home. I took the part-time job. I told him it was important that nobody on the dock knew he was my uncle. I didn't want any special treatment or the workers acting different around me—knowing the foreman was my uncle. Back then, families took care of each other in such ways. Those people who worked on the dock were never informed that Fred was my relative.

Working there, the wind blew so hard it seemed like it was going to cut me into pieces. I wore two or three sweaters, a jacket, two pair of pants and a mask on my face. The other workers called me the "Masked Man." After closing the barber shop, I would go to the loading docks at 6 pm and work until 11:30 pm. For five hours each night, I moved merchandise from the loading docks on to the trucks. All the loading of the big boxes was done by hand. I loaded the back of the trucks and another guy loaded the front.

One night, I was leaving the loading dock, and I went to start my car but it wouldn't start. Then I heard a loud "POP." The temperature read 12 degrees below zero. I thought to myself: "Oh Boy." I decided to quit that Job. I felt that my wife and my kids would rather have me alive than dead from the exhausting cold.

After 13 years of marriage, Rosemary and I still had never taken a day of vacation, and she never let on like she was disappointed. She never complained that her cousins went on vacations—not once. Then, I got a brainstorm. I knew I wanted to take her some place special. So, I planned a trip to a vacation spot in Wisconsin about 70 miles away. It was a hotel resort called The Schwartz House, and we finally took first our vacation that year. The Schwartz House gave us meals. They also took our kids out on tours.

Before I left on vacation, I decided to put a sign on the window of my shop that read: "John is going on vacation for 12 days," and the sign had the dates I was to be gone. Before I went on vacation, the shop got a little bit more crowded. My regulars came in and some of them gave me a couple extra bucks and said: "Enjoy your vacation." Having a couple extra couple bucks, in those days, was considered good money.

When I came back from vacation, business got better. The customers I had lost returned in the following weeks. I thought if taking a vacation worked this well, then, next year, I would try two weeks. My mother-in-law often offered to take care of the kids if we wanted to do something alone, so, we took her up on her offer the following year. In 1974, we took two weeks driving around on a vacation—just the two of us, Rosemary and I enjoyed our own vacation.

Once I found out that the customers were so faithful, I started taking a little more vacation time each year. Year after year, I put a sign on the shop window that read: "John is going on vacation—from a certain date to a certain date." Each year it kept me very busy at the shop the week before and the week after our vacations. If I ever lost a customer, I would get a new one in his place, or my customers who went away would come back later. That's the way it always worked out. I did that for years. Then the neighborhood changed.

DOs & TABOOs

DO: *Some people like to play the ponies. In those days, apart from baseball, betting the horses was a favorite sport for many people.*

TABOO: *There is a right and wrong place for everything. My business was no place to let a bookie make his bets.*

DO: *Taking part-time jobs is a good way to get ahead with finances or make extra money.*

TABOO: *It's not ok to work side jobs in weather that is 12 degrees below zero when you could lose your life and leave your wife and children without a father.*

CHAPTER FOUR

Our Orland Park Home And
My Second Barber Shop

I reached a stage when my lifestyle kept growing. I moved up in a higher social class and bought a new home and a second barber shop.

The barber business made it possible for me to meet all kinds of people. I made more new friends. I met Rosemary and became part of her family, and of course, it gave me everything I needed to buy a home and support my own family. The business gave me a good position the community, a good reputation and a lifetime of memories.

In the 1976 desegregation era, the City of Chicago started busing children around to different schools, Rosemary and I decided to sell our home in the Chicago inter-city on LaPorte, and buy a new home in the Orland Park suburbs in 1977. The first two weeks of school, my son Robert went to stay in our newly built Orland Park home all alone—so he could attend his first two weeks of classes in his new school. The name of the school was Sandburg High School. It was considered a number-one-rated high school in the Chicago suburbs during those days. There was literally no one else in the subdivision accept him. Robert was the first person to move into the area because none of the other homes had even been built yet. Each day, the bus picked him up in the morning before school and then brought him back home at night.

I recall the Sandburg school bus drivers were very strict. If the kids made too much noise while riding on the bus, the driver would turn the bus around and go back to the school until they learned to ride quietly and respectfully.

When our kids got a little bigger, of course, we had to watch them a little closer. We made sure that they always completed their homework. Rosemary always looked after them in a caring and loving way. She usually handled the kids, and she did a great job.

My youngest son, John, would often complete his homework during school hours so he didn't have to do it after school. That way when he got home he was allowed free time. The school teachers were satisfied even if the homework was completed during school hours—as long as it was completed properly. Both of my boys earned pretty good grades and were pretty good in school.

Once, I bought a Moped scooter for my son John. Within a couple of weeks, the police showed up at the front door, because they had stopped him for driving the scooter on the street without a driver's license. We viewed the scooter as a bicycle with a motor. The police viewed it as a motor vehicle. It never dawned on us that he could be cited for driving on the streets without a driver's license, so I ended up using the scooter myself to zip around from place to place.

To understand the description and utility of the Moped scooter, one needs to go back to the early days of the bicycle and the invention that revolutionized the 20th century—the internal combustion engine. Inventers mounted a small combustion engine on a bicycle and presto, they had the Moped Scooter (Motor+PEDals). It was the precursor of all motorcycles. Pedals were used on all Mopeds—used both as a starter device and as emergency fallback on human power. (Wikipedia)

It wasn't long before I had an accident on the scooter when a back tire blew out. I broke my leg and my arm. I also took a bad gash to my head. I was off work for a while, after the Moped accident. One day, I was sitting outside the front of our home when a neighbor who lived just down the street walked by and asked me what had happened. He stood out front on the sidewalk talking with me until I invited him to come up to the house and sit with me and talk. He told me his name was Julius Hinton. He was a black man. We became very good friends that day. I think because he was black that many people treated him as though he was part of different group of people. But he and his family were our neighbors; and from that day forward, they were always invited to all of our neighborhood get-togethers and were considered friends in the neighborhood. In our neighborhood, I didn't see any racial stuff take place. To this day, I still get greeting cards from Julius on every occasion.

After we lived in Orland Park for a couple of years, we started giving a lot of thought about Rosemary's parents, who were getting older. They were living in Oak Park—about 20 miles away. Rosemary and I decided to buy second house two doors down on our same street. We decided to buy the house just in case Frank and Adeline were to ever get sick. We thought it would put us in a position that we could care for them if needed. It was even more convenient because there was a hospital about three miles away from our home. The house was a fair price. I had a good connection with the bank. So, we bought it and moved them in.

Holidays with our families were very important times for celebration. We always felt that holidays were for the family. Christmas was the most important holiday. We always spent Christmas with Rosemary's parents until Adeline got to the age when she could no longer cook and do things for our celebrations. Rosemary then took over all such things, then Frank and Adeline started joining us for holidays.

We always went to mass on Christmas and Easter. Being Catholic, we always ate fish on Friday. It was a Catholic tradition then. So we always prepared a dinner of fish. The meal usually consisted of fish, pasta, and broccoli.

One of our favorite traditional breakfasts was called: "Frittata." It was an Italian dish with Italian sausage, Ricotta cheese, Mozzarella cheese, and eggs. The ingredients were all fried together and looked like a big fat pancake when it was ready to serve. Rosemary usually prepared these breakfasts on both Christmas and Easter.

On Christmas mornings, I usually started the day with my first cup of coffee, and the kids spent the time opening gifts. Then, we would all dress up for Christmas Mass. It was the same on Easter. Holiday celebrations with my family made me very happy.

I was at my West side barber shop for more than eight years. Then, I opened a second barber shop on the South side of Chicago, in Brian Park. My first idea was to find a barber shop closer to home. I eventually found one on Archer Avenue named *Archer Avenue Barber Shop*. I liked it, but at same the time, I felt it was a little too small. I moved into the shop. Later, I was talking with a neighbor, who was also a barber, about the situation. He asked me why I didn't want it. I told him I thought I wanted something bigger. He suggested I stay there for the time being, and if I found one a little bigger, then I could sell the small one and move into a bigger one. So, I told him: "I think you're right." I stayed.

I changed the name to *John's Barber Shop* so I wouldn't lose my long-time customers, and I closed the West side shop. I ended up staying in that small barber shop for more than thirty years. It was on a good street. We had car dealers close by, and there were a lot of other people living in the area—all who needed haircuts. It was profitable to stay.

The area was a mixture of Polish and Italians. I always felt it was a "Hell of good neighborhood." Everybody in the area would give a lot. Everybody went to church. At that time, I had one customer who was with me for thirty years. When I left Chicago, some of my customers, who came with me from my first shop, ended up staying with me for more than forty years.

There was a detectives department near my new barber shop. The Detective Commander was named John Berge. He would send his other detectives to my new barber shop to get their haircuts. It created a very respectable clientele. I was well-liked and I had a good reputation with them.

After twenty years of shaving and cutting himself every morning, a man from the detective department decided he had had enough. He told me he wanted me to start shaving him. He came not knowing I was active in the in the Catholic Church.

I told him: I would give him a close razor shave, but I would be easy on him and shave him with a little "grace." I finished shaving him and said: "That will be ten dollars." The detective thought my price was a bit high, but he paid the bill and went to work.

The next morning he looked in the mirror, and his face was just as smooth as it was when he left my shop the day before. Not bad, he thought. At least I don't need to pay for a shave every day. The next morning, his face was still smooth. Two days later, the detective's face was still smooth.

It was more than he could take, so he returned to my barber shop and said: "I thought ten dollars was a high price for a shave, but it's been four days and my whiskers still haven't started growing back." The expression on my face didn't even change, I just responded: "You were shaved with a little "Grace": *'Once Shaved—always Shaved.'*" (Anonymous)

The guy that sold me the first barber shop gave me some words of advice. They are words I go by even today:

He told me: "In poor things, what you can't do with your hands—do with your mouth." In other words, he said, "If you can't please them by giving them a haircut, then talk to them with a smile. Just try to convince them, in your own language, that what you did is not the worst thing in the world. Then, on the other hand if you please them, you've got it made. If you can't please them, you only have to go through that for fifteen minutes—once."

I found, if I can't please them they won't come back. If I lose one customer, I'll get another. And it really worked out that way. Some customers might say John's not the best barber in the world, but he has a hell of a good sense of humor.

I have had customers that would come in time after time and say: "John, I want this or I want that. I had already given them one half-dozen haircuts, but for some reason, they wanted to tell me again and again.

For example: I had a customer named Poshinski. He worked as a Post Master. I must have given him haircuts for 25 years. He would come into the shop and each time he would say: "John, I want this. I want that. I want the other." Each time, I answered: "Alright." But one time he came in and made it half way through the haircut before he started telling me what he wanted done to his hair.

I said: "Mr. Poshinski, you blew it! Because, if you didn't say anything, I was going to give you a free haircut—because it was the first time that you didn't say: 'Give me this or give me that'—I was going to tell you: 'Mr. Poshinski, since you didn't say anything, I'm giving you a haircut on the house.' But, you blew it. I apologize."

Mr. Poshinski said: "Next time, I'll keep my mouth shut."

I told him: "Next time it won't do you any good."

We both laughed. That's the kind of stuff I put up with in a barber shop. And, I had to take it with a good sense of humor, because it's not worth it to get aggravated. It's only ten or fifteen minutes of work. Since I've heard those words of advice, I think I've done a hell-of a-nice-job!

One of my customers came into the shop complaining about his job—saying: "Today, my job was a 'pain-in-the-ass.' But, on the other hand, he said, I thank God that I have a job." He told me: "John, you have it made. No one ever tells you what to do."

Thirty seconds later, he said, "John, take a little bit more hair off the top and off the back. And, shave my neck."

So then I returned the favor by telling him: "You thought I have it made—and now you tell me what to do!" So, the reality is: Barbers take orders from everyone who walks in and sits in the barber chairs.

One of my customers would come for his haircuts. And, from time to time, he would bring along his seven-year-old son, Brian. Each time I gave the boy a haircut, the child was a pain—*where the sun don't shine!* The father would politely ask the boy: "Please be still so John can cut your hair."

I finally got fed up with the boy's nonsense and asked the father to take a walk. I told him: "Brian and I will work it out."

As the father walked out the door, I asked Brian, "Do you see this big strap? It is the strap that I use to sharpen the razors. If you don't sit still and let me cut your hair, I will make your butt black and blue. So Brian, be still, because a haircut only takes ten minutes."

The father returned to see his young son sitting in the chair like a little gentleman. And, after that, each time Brian came into the barber shop, he was a perfect little gentleman and a good customer. Sometimes, you just have to show kids—who is BOSS. That day Brian grew up a little, and it took a barber shop setting to help him grow.

I was always pleased with my customers. They continued coming back. They usually walked out and thanked me. The money has always been good. But, when I saw customers walk out with a smile, it always meant a lot more.

When the long-hair came in, the high-class hair stylists came in with it. The hair stylists were making big-big money. I felt the financial crunch; but people said: "John, just hang on to your shop." There were factories on both sides of us, so I hung around. Later, short hair came back in and the long hair went back out. Those high-class hair stylists couldn't stick around. People were still paying me eight to nine dollars instead of paying them fifteen dollars, so the hair stylists went away, and my business got even better. As far as barber shops and hair salons come and go, the area became like a ghost town. Later there was just me and one other barber 1-1/2 miles away.

The amount I was paying for rent at the barber shop on Archer Avenue started at 80 dollars per month. The last month's rent was 280 dollars per month (34 years later). Everybody else, including the high-class hair salons, ended up paying 600 to 650 dollars per month.

Because I was there for such a long time, my landlord of 20 years only raised the rent five dollars here and ten dollars there. He would leave the keys to the building in the barber shop with me. So, when people came to look at the-vacancies in the complex, he would just tell them: "Go see John the Barber and he will let you in." If the people liked the open shops, they would bring back their application to see what kind of deal the landlord could make with them. By the time I left there, in 1996, haircuts were about 10 or 11 dollars.

After Robert graduated from high school, he decided he wanted to become a Priest in the Catholic Church. At the time it seemed to Rosemary and to me like one of the most important things in our world—to have a son who chose the life of an Ordained Priest.

It didn't turn out that way.

When Robert was finished with the Nile College of Priesthood, he came to us and told us he no longer had the calling. So, he changed his major, after four years of college, and he went into teaching. Looking back, the investment we made in his education didn't seem to do much good. We learned to not put too much hope on our expectations.

Then, he changed his mind again and went to a different college to become a Human Resource Director making big money in downtown Chicago. Later, he gave up on that career too. Since then, he has been teaching for the past 14 years. He met his wife and was married. They have three children. On the face they seem to have a very nice family.

DOs & TABOOs

DO: It's ok to come into my barber shop and let me know the things you want done to your hair—perhaps even for the first five or six times.

TABOO: After that, it is important to remember two things. (1) You might be giving up a free haircut, and (2) don't forget, I still have the razor strap.

DO: It's great to buy your son a Moped scooter to zip around the neighborhood.

TABOO: Don't let him ride the scooter until he has a driver's license, because the police might show up at your front door.

Worse than that, The scooter could turn out to be such a temptation that, like me, you might take it out for a spin and end up in the hospital ten days with a broken arm, broken leg, and a hole in your head.

Chapter Five

Moving To Arizona

Our in-laws were getting older and our boys were nearly grown up. Around that time, Adeline came up with an idea that we thought was goofy: She said she wanted to go and live in Arizona. We thought she was losing it.

The first thoughts I had when I heard Adeline wanted to go to Arizona was how the temperature gets as high as 110 degrees—and how it could kill us. We couldn't even stand 90-degree temperatures in Chicago. But Rosemary told me that 110 degrees in Arizona is better than 90 degrees in Chicago because the humidity in Arizona is so much lower. So, Rosemary and I decided to take a vacation to Arizona.

We came to Arizona in May to visit Rosemary's uncle Fred who had already moved to Sun Village, which is in the City of Surprise. We stayed ten days in Arizona and then we went on to Las Vegas. While we were visiting Fred, he showed us some really nice homes in the area.

One thing that sold me about buying a home in Arizona was the small amount of property taxes. By comparison, property taxes were about 4000 dollars in Chicago compared to 800 dollars we would have to pay in Arizona. The only thing that was more expensive in Arizona was the automobile registration fees. So I suggested to Rosemary that maybe we should buy a winter home in Arizona. She took me up on it.

One night in bed, Rosemary asked me a question: "Are we going to do it?" At first I thought she was talking about being intimate, but what she was referring to was: "Are we going to buy a house in Arizona." Our first thought was to buy a second home so we could come spend the winter months in Arizona.

We made an offer on a house, but the offer was declined. So we went back to Chicago. Then on Labor Day, we came back out and stayed in a 125-dollar-per-week condo by the Sun Dome in Sun City West. We left Chicago in 90-degree weather and when we arrived in Arizona it was over 100 degrees, but the Arizona heat felt a lot better.

The first thing I told Rosemary was: "I think we are going to die in such heat." But a couple of days later, the heat started feeling really good. That Labor Day weekend, we bought our first Arizona home in Sun Village.

In October, Rosemary took three days and brought her parents, Frank and Adeline, to Arizona to stay in assisted living.

In November, Rosemary moved to our new Sun Village home.

In December, I came out to Arizona two weeks before Christmas to spend a few weeks with Rosemary and her cousins, Pat, Rose and their husbands.

During that time, Frank was in a coma. I was originally planning to return to Chicago on January 7, but Frank passed away. Adeline was still in assisted living, and I ended up flying Adeline and Rosemary back to Chicago, and we laid Frank to rest. After we laid Frank to rest, Rosemary and Adeline came back to Arizona. I stayed in Chicago until March to settle our affairs.

In Chicago, I belonged to the local chapter of the Holy Name Society for many years. The people in the Society found out that I was moving to Arizona. Soon after, a reporter from the Brian Park local neighborhood newspaper told me they wanted to write a little story about the time I worked in Brian Park. I said OK because I lived there for 30 years. I was well treated by them too. I told the reporter that it was time to move on and why we chose to move to Arizona. I explained that I had a problem with the cold winters in Chicago.

One of the members of the Holy Name Society decided to throw me a surprise-going-away-party. They usually held their meetings on the second Thursday of the month. Knowing that I closed the barber shop at 3 pm, he asked me to come to their Thursday meeting after I get off of work—just to say goodbye to the gang. He didn't say it was a surprise get-together for me. He just said it would probably be my last meeting there. At first, I wasn't planning to go. I explained that I usually closed the barber shop at 3 pm and that I really didn't feel like sticking around for four hours until 7 pm.

Then he asked me again: "Oh—just this one time—"c'mon'!"

I answered: "This time I will try to make it."

Then on Saturday the Priest from our church told me he found out that I was moving to Arizona. I told him that I was taking the opportunity to move to Arizona. I explained that my wife was already there with her cousins who were also planning to move out West. I told him: "We just decided to do it," and that I was leaving March 1. He also suggested that I come to the meeting on Thursday. So, at 3 pm I closed the shop and walked around mall until about 6:45 pm, and then I went to the meeting.

The meeting was on their second floor. When I walked up the stairs, some cameras started flashing and a movie camera started running. The guy who greeted me at the door said: "John, this little get-together we're having tonight is for you." At first I didn't believe him, but then everyone came up to me and greeted me and wished me a happy trip. It made me very happy.

They all came together saying: "Thank you, John, for being such a nice person in our neighborhood." Many of those people lived there for 50 to 60 years. Many were old timers. I gave most of them haircuts, and I had also given haircuts to their sons and even their grandsons. That is how long my history in the neighborhood spanned.

I finally put my barber shop up for sale. The only advertising I did was when I went to the barber supply-house. I told the man at the front desk that I planned to sell my barber shop for 2000 dollars. A day later, a young man called me to tell me he was interested. He came to the shop and gave me a 500-dollar down payment and said he wanted to return the next day to pick everything up. I told him he would have to wait until the following Saturday. I wanted to finish out the week—saying goodbye to customers.

On Saturday, he came to pick up the barber equipment which included two 150-year-old barber chairs, a back bar and mirror, six waiting chairs, a cash register, a show case, the neon sign that read: *John's Barber Shop* and the barber pole from outside. While he was there to pick up the equipment, he also bought my air conditioning system, a small refrigerator, a microwave oven and the old recliner that I used to take naps and read magazines when business was slow.

The young man used the equipment to open an old style barber shop in the prestigious Palmer House. Chicago's Palmer House was a historical high-class hotel with fancy restaurants—where businesses held conventions and presidential candidates gave speeches.

The theme for the young man's new shop was: *The Old Class Barber Shop.*

When my shop closed and all my affairs were settled in Chicago, I packed up the remainder of our personal items and came out West to join Rosemary in Sun Village.

After about four years in Sun Village, Rosemary and I went out for a Sunday morning breakfast, and afterwards we looked at some model homes in the area. We decided to go into the models, and a gentleman took us for a ride in the subdivision of Mountain Vista Ranch. He told us we would have our pick of lots—considering we would be one of the first to buy a home in the new subdivision. As it turned out, it would be our last home together.

The home has the best view out on the back patio—where a person can see for miles and miles. The Western sky has the most beautiful sunsets. Both old and new friends in Surprise would come to our home to enjoy meals and get-togethers. I often made the sauce for the spaghetti and our friends brought sausage or salads or different dishes. We spent many evenings or weekends together shooting the breeze. We created the same kind of friendly atmosphere we enjoyed so much in Chicago.

Five years after we moved to Arizona, Rosemary and I decided to go on vacation to Italy to visit my sister Ida. Robert went with us. A few days after Labor Day 2001 we left on our trip. After we arrived in the Tenuta Village, about 9:00 am, we heard news of the terrorist attacks on New York City's World Trade Center, the U.S. Pentagon and Flight 93 in Pennsylvania—a flight thwarted by passengers—which many believe was intended to destroy the White House.

Being in Italy during the 9-11 attacks was a tremendous scare for us, because the entire world's airline system was shut down. We didn't know when we would get to leave to go back to America. There were so many things to consider such as getting home or whether or not the United States was going to war. It brought up a lot of memories from my childhood when my father faced a similar situation, and it took him almost seven months to get back to our homeland.

Fortunately, we were able to make our original flight on time; however, ninety days later, the United States was at war in Afghanistan. Our country declared world-wide military response against terrorism and the leader of Al-Qaida, Osama Bin Laden (believed to be the master-mind of the 9-11 attacks). It took almost ten years before American Special Forces—Navy Seals killed him. It took way too long for justice to come, but I don't think we should let our guard down just because he is dead. There are still a lot of hateful terrorists who want Americans to die. Today all we have done is cut off the head the snake—but it (Al-Qaida) is still alive.

Once we made it back home, things eventually turned back to normal. Some mornings, we would sit on our front porch on a little breakfast table and read the newspaper and enjoy our small breakfasts together.

About three years after we moved to Arizona, I bought Rosemary a nice organ. She enjoyed playing it very much. The organ was a hardwood three-board-key Kendall. We kept it in our den across the room from her computer.

On Sundays, we always went to Mass. There were times when we went out for Sunday breakfast at small restaurants or to the Elks lodge—invited as guests of our friends and then came home to read the Sunday newspaper, and Rosemary played the organ. While she played the organ, most of the time, I would doze off for little power naps.

After we moved to Surprise, Rosemary started working for three days per week. I enjoyed helping her out on those days, so she could come home and enjoy the rest of her day. We always enjoyed cooking and cleaning the kitchen together.

One Friday night, I was helping with the laundry, and Rosemary caught me folding the cloths while they were still damp. She didn't like the way damp cloths looked later when she pulled them out of the drawer, so when she realized what I had done, she said, "Tenuta, I'm going to ship you back to Chicago." That's the worst she ever got. She never made a big deal or drama out of anything.

We had a way of being playful with each other.

One day while we were returning home to Sun Village, we drove up to the back entrance to our gated-community. I asked her if she would get out of the car and open the gate. I handed her the gate-key. She got out and walked around the car and opened the gate.

When she got back in the car, she was quiet. It took her a while before she realized what I had done, but when I parked the car in our garage, she said: "You have a lot of nerve—making me get out of the car—when you could have opened the gate from your window. "YOU MADE ME DO IT." That was the kind of playful nature we had with each other.

I stayed home a lot. Eventually, I told Rosemary: "I am not going to stay at home all the time and live a prisoner in my own home again—I've got to do something—even if I go to work in a grocery store, I have to get a job."

So, I went to one of the barber shops in the area of Surprise, and one of the barbers there recommended that I go to the Arizona Barber Board to get a barber's license in Arizona.

The Barber Board told me if I was from Indiana, they could honor my existing Barber's license and re-license me in Arizona, but since my license was from Illinois, they could not honor it. I'm still not sure why they could honor a license from Indiana, but not a license from Illinois.

I told them: "You guys discriminate." I exclaimed, "I have been a barber all my life, and now you tell me I can't be a barber in Arizona unless I go to school. It doesn't seem right. I didn't even go to school when I was a kid, and you expect me to go to school at 63 years old?"

One nice gentleman there explained how we could get around the problem. He said, "I'll give you a phone number in Arkansas. You call the number and they will send you an application from Arkansas. You fill it out and provide them proof of your license from Illinois, and they will send you a license from Arkansas. You come back here with your Arkansas license and we can honor it and give you a license here. I called the Arkansas Board and they sent me an application.

I sent the application in and waited one week, then two weeks, then three weeks, and finally, when three weeks were up, I called and talked to the Arkansas Board. I explained to them: "I am John Tenuta. I live in Arizona. I sent you an application for a license from Arkansas." They told me my application arrived in their mail the day before. So a week later, the license from Arkansas showed up at my home. I took that Arkansas license to the Arizona Barber Board. They looked it over and asked for my life history.

I showed them all my Illinois licenses and said; "Here are my licenses from Illinois. Pick any one you want from 1953 on." The man answered: "Mr. Tenuta, give us your birth date, your Arizona address and 80 bucks." I gave him the information and the money, and he gave me a license. Why they didn't do that with my Illinois license—I don't know. Now, I just renew the license every two years. I have worked in Arizona for nearly 14 years now—two days per week.

Working in barber shops is a little different in Arizona. Some the barbers provide different services to bring in new customers. One barber I worked for also sold gold.

In one barber shop, a really good-looking girl was giving a man a manicure.

"How about a date when you finish work?" the man asked.

"I can't," she replied, "I am married."

"So, call up your husband and tell him you're going to visit a sick girlfriend," said the man.

"Why don't you tell him yourself." said the girl, "He's the one shaving you." (Anonymous)

I always renew my barber's license by mailing them the check with my license number attached in January. But, four years ago, I waited until after my birthday in February; I sent it in late near the beginning of March. They sent it back. They told me they wanted my birth certificate. So, I called them and asked what happened. One of the Barber Board officers explained that there are so many aliens in Arizona—who just come for the license, and are not born here, that they have to investigate each case before they give out new licenses. I finally got a copy of my birth certificate and sent them the money, and I got another license.

Finally Rosemary and I were both working and keeping ourselves busy and happy in Arizona. We lived in the Mountain Vista Ranch home for six years before she went back to Orland Park for medical treatment. As it turned out, it was the last time we actually lived together before she passed away.

When she left for Chicago, I told Rosemary, that I would save her place in the bedroom, and I would not sleep there again until she returns.

DOs & TABOOs

DO: *Looking back, it was lucky when we found Rosemary the Kendall organ, because we both got so much enjoyment from her playing it. She loved playing and I loved listening.*

TABOOs: *It was not so good to snooze off too many times while she was playing, because, for Rosemary, it was also fun playing on her computer—and out went the Sunday morning music.*

CHAPTER SIX

Looking Back Over Great Times In Life.

I still get new customers who come in for haircuts and talk with me as though they have known me for years. I respect the new friendships. I have considered retiring but, after talking to most of my customers, they tell me: "No." They say that I am still a young boy. The most important thing is that I still enjoy my life as a barber. I think for now, it's a good idea to keep on cutting hair, because it keeps me occupied and keeps me in touch with my friends.

The most important thing in work is: Whatever kind of work I am doing, I have to enjoy my work. If I were to go to work with a chip on my shoulder, it would not be good for my health.

As far as my relationship with Rosemary went, the one thing I appreciated most was how we always knew what each other was doing and where each other was at. We spent our life together like *ONE*.

In forty-five years of marriage, I don't think she went grocery shopping more than three times alone. Once in a great while I would suggest: "Why don't you just go?" She would just reply: "You don't have anything to do—we'll both go." So I always went with her.

I would regularly get home about one half hour after I closed the barber shop. We didn't have a phone in the car, but I had one at the shop. If I had a customer who came in a little late, then, I would get home about 15 minutes later, and I would always call first to let her know.

Most of the time, I would cheat the clock and try to get off work a little early. When I got home, Rosemary usually had dinner waiting for me. Whenever I went somewhere, I always let her know the time I planned to be home.

Honesty was the most important thing in our marriage. We were like two buddies. If she had to go somewhere, then I would take her. And then I would go pick her up. If she wanted to drive, then she would drive. Rosemary never felt like she needed the freedom to go here or there alone. We loved being together. We were like one. The type of closeness we enjoyed doesn't work for all couples, but it was perfect for us.

It was the same way with our kids—they didn't feel they needed to have all kinds of different games just to keep up with the other kids. Kids nowadays seem to want so many things—even my own grandchildren think they want everything. It's a different world we live in today.

Life when I grew up and when I raised my own family was all about the home, the family and being together. When we all got home—including the kids, we enjoyed staying with each other. Other men I knew liked to go out to the bars and clubs. I remember a time when I was 18 or 19 years old, I couldn't wait until I would turn 21 years old, because then I could go out to the bars. It didn't happen that way. It seems like whenever I walked past the bars, the smell of cigarettes and booze smelled terrible to me. I knew it just wasn't my kind of entertainment.

I was never a heavy drinker. Occasionally I would drink a glass of beer. Once in a while, I would have a glass of wine. When I did drink, the kids and my wife would kid around with me and say: "Watch out, tonight there is going to be trouble." Now the doctor tells me that a little glass of wine—perhaps a little white Zinfandel or Vin-Rose is ok.

When I went home, I always had somebody waiting for me. When Rosemary went to work, I drove her, and then I picked her up. Once in a while, we stopped to get something to eat, just for a change. Sometimes, we just wanted some junk food.

When I finally found a barber shop I liked, I started enjoying my work in Arizona.

A man came into the barber shop and saw a sign our wall that read: *Shaves that will last one year for 150 dollars.*

The man took me up on the special deal. I shaved him and then I rubbed a special after-shave lotion on his face and he went home.

The next morning, the man got up, showered, and while he was drying off, he noticed he had a regular day of growth on his cheeks.

So, he came back to the barber shop and asked me: "What happened to my one-year shave?"

I asked the man: "Sir, what did you do when you woke up in the morning?"

He said: "I woke up and took a shower."

I explained: "You washed off the magic after shave lotion. But if you want, I will give you another deal for half price. For 75 dollars, I'll give you a shave that will last six months."

The man left. (Anonymous)

One day, Rosemary took the car to do some shopping in Surprise while I was at work. She planned to pick me up at 4:30 pm, but I got off about one-half hour early, so I started walking South toward home in hopes that I could head her off on her way to pick me up. But, she didn't see me because she was driving looking intently straight forward—not expecting me to be on the side of the road.

She missed me again when she passed me on her way back home. Then she returned to the barber shop and missed me a third time. Finally, when she arrived back home the second time, she caught up to me at the back gate of our community. I ended up walking about three miles in 110-degree heat wearing a shirt and tie. When she saw me, she said: *"GET IN THE FRICKIN' CAR!"* I think that day she was a little hotter than me.

Right up until today, guys come in to get a haircut, and we still exchange stories about our lives. Often times it was me doing the talking.

Many times, my customers have suggested that I write a book about my life. Not being able to write very well, I set out to find someone who would write the book as I tell my story. So now at 77 years old, I am producing my book—even without an education.

I have a lot of memories about the things I have done in my life and the things that I am proud about. But looking back, the thing that I am most pleased with is how Rosemary came into my life. She was the most precious thing—that ever happened to me.

Looking back, I feel most troubled about the how American's people are losing trust in government and the how with each new president, it seems to get worse.

During the President Johnson Administration, the country went through a lot of unrest. The military draft was activated and the country was deep-seated into a war in Viet Nam. It was often called the Black War.

Thousands of young Americans—usually poor and uneducated were being drafted into the armed forces. The war divided the country. Few people understood why the United States was at war in Southeast Asia. Our people were being told the war was to stop communism. I feel the reality was that the war was just an economic way of keeping Americans employed by making the machines of war.

There were riots around the country protesting the war in Viet Nam. Kent State University experienced a riot where the National Guard took up arms against students who were protesting for peace. Young men left the country to avoid getting drafted. They were labeled Draft Dodgers and scorned by many of the American people. Young Americans argued that the Viet Nam War was not a vital interest for the United States.

DOs & TABOOs

DO: *It is ok to walk and try to head someone off if they are coming to pick you up. It's better to first let the person know.*

TABOO: *It's not ok when you end up walking in 110-degree weather because you could like me end up walking for three miles—scaring the hell out of your wife and getting her madder than you've ever seen her. Because right then, even if you tell her that she looked so good driving the nice clean car, she might not respond with a mile-long-smile. The smile might take a while.*

CHAPTER SEVEN

Presidents And The Economy

I came to America at a time when people believed in the leaders and the laws of the land. Anyone who had a dream could come here and make their dreams come true.

Now there is so much skepticism that teachers even plant ideas in students' minds that America never landed on the moon. There are also stories out there that George W. Bush orchestrated the 9/11 attacks in order to create the war in Afghanistan. People are so skeptical about anything coming from news that our citizens don't know what to think or who to believe.

Kids are so caught up in wanting to be popular that they pay 500 dollars—a price of a used car—for a pair of basketball shoes in order to be "Like Mike."

Today, it seems that the people who are running the country are focused on the wrong things. The country doesn't seem to be focused on helping our own people like they did when I came here.

When I came here, in 1952, America was the land of opportunity. Anybody could do something to make a buck. The things that were required were that people respected you and you respected them. It was a place where friendships and trust were born. Neighbors were helping each other. They would get together in the evenings outdoors in the humidity and form strong bonds by talking into the middle of the night sometimes. It seems that when the air-conditioners came in; that way of life started slowing down because people quit going out in the evening as much.

Looking back over my life, it seems like many of the country's values, which I based my own high-hopes on have changed.

To start, I came to America five months before Dwight Eisenhower was elected as the President of the United States. The country was still rebounding from World War II. At that time, the United States was considered the strongest nation on Earth. The country had power, jobs and money. Anyone who wanted to work could find a job. More importantly, anyone who wanted to become a business-owner had a great chance for success. From the time I arrived in America, it only took nine years to become a homeowner and business owner. I never had a problem finding work or even side-work whenever I wanted extra money.

It was reasonable to think that with a little structure in my budget that I could also make money by investing. Thirteen years after I was married, Rosemary and I had saved enough money and built enough equity in our home to place a handsome down payment on an investment property. Then we eventually created more savings from that investment than we did from my full time job as a barber.

Once a person established a line credit, there was always a bank or lending institution competing for his business investment opportunities. Also, during that time, the U.S. economy was largely based on people who were buying a new car on credit every two years. I never bought into that idea. Instead, Rosemary and I were determined to be liquid with our assets, and we paid cash for almost everything we owned.

Silver dollars were made of silver. Quarters, dimes and half dollars were also made of silver. It was common to see ten-, five-, and one-dollar bills that had seals on them that read redeemable in gold or silver in circulation. They were called Gold and Silver Certificates. The silver coins and certificates began to disappear. Once I was at the grocery store, and a lady shopper in front of me paid her bill with a one-dollar silver certificate. The grocery store cashier took the silver certificate and put it in her own pocket and paid the woman's grocery bill with a standard one dollar bill.

Since then, the country and economy seems to have lost that old image. Jobs have consistently been disappearing and going overseas. Technology has cost the uneducated workers many jobs. If I had come to America during this era, I don't how I would have succeeded as well as I did.

One day, a customer came into the barber shop and told how he had closed his second-generation business because of changing times. He told me that he closed it the week before. He said that his business provided a good wage, health insurance, vacation pay, Christmas bonuses and retirement benefits. It wasn't good enough.

The week before, his workers decided to join the Union and insisted they get higher pay. While the workers were picketing outside the front of his store, he called the agency that rented him the equipment and asked them to come get it and take it away from the back entrance of his shop. Once the equipment was completely removed, he opened his front door and allowed the workers to come in the shop. They came in and discovered there was no longer any equipment or any place to work at their trade. My customer told me he was forced to make that decision to close up his shop. That was why he was there in the barber shop loafing around with me. He had already earned enough to retire, so the pressure the labor union put on his company forced him to close. The people who lost out were the workers who bought into the idea of the Union way.

The next day, a customer came into our barber shop. He sat down in the chair, and one of our barbers cut his hair. After the barber was done, the customer got up and took out his money.

Right then, he noticed the barber went over and peed in the corner of the barber shop.

The barber finished and came back.

As the barber came back, the customer said: "Listen, it's none of my business, but why would you piss in the corner of your own barber shop?"

The barber said, "Hey, my lease is up in two weeks. Why should I care?"

The barber went over to the cash register and rang up the haircut. He came back with the man's change, and the customer was squatting down crapping on the floor.

The barber said: "What the heck are you doing?"

The customer answered, "What the hell do I care? I'm leaving now!" (Anonymous)

Technology has also taken away a lot of jobs from Americans. Now there are robots overseas doing the work on our automobiles that were once done by American workers. Cars are made to last longer, so there is no longer a stable economy based solely on people buying a new car every two years.

Careers are such that people move from job to job for higher pay rather than build a reputation of being good dependable tradesmen. Most of our kids are educated and they don't want to do hard work, so laborers from other countries come to America to do the jobs that our teenagers once did for summer jobs—like landscaping, dishwashing, car washing and grocery store helpers and on and on and on.

Now many Americans are over educated and can't find work in their field of choice they were trained in because many illegal immigrants get free education and work at their jobs for far less money.

The deterioration of the country's image, in my opinion, started with the people losing their faith in the presidential office during the President Nixon administration.

Real mistrust started when Richard Nixon then became president. To many, his greatest legacy was ending the terrible war in Viet Nam. Then, as our soldiers returned to the States, they were labeled Baby-Killers and War Mongers by those young Americans who protested the war. Many came back home wounded for life and addicted to drugs. Over 50 thousand soldiers died in Viet Nam.

During the Nixon's presidency, the Vice President was ousted for income tax evasion. Then, Nixon himself got caught lying to the American people in the Watergate cover-up scandal which caused him to be the first President to ever resign from office.

Then, Gerald Ford, Nixon's second Vice President, took Nixon's place as President for just a short term after President Nixon resigned. Ford was not re-elected.

Jimmy Carter was elected as President, but he lost favor because of his mixed messages of diplomacy. In one of the greatest acts of American diplomacy in U.S. history, President Carter pardoned all the draft dodgers who had fled to Canada and other countries. On the other hand, the diplomatic measures he used in the Iranian Hostage Crisis cost him a second term in office.

The Iranian hostage crisis was when fifty Americans were held hostage in Iran for 444 days. Carter was considered a weak president because he avoided another war. By the time his presidency ended, the world saw the United States as losing its strength, because Iranian crisis also exposed the U.S. military equipment as obsolete when he sent seven helicopters into Iran and they all crashed because they weren't built to fly in dry and sandy desert conditions.

Ronald Regan was sworn in as the next elected President. The night President Regan was signed into office, the Iranians released the hostages. Regan came into office and stimulated the American image by rebuilding the American military and the national infrastructure. Even though the world saw Regan as a powerful President, it was the American farmer who suffered because under his administration, the American bankers made billions of dollars available to the American farmer and encouraged the farmers to grow wheat from fence to fence to supply the Soviet Union wheat and grain during the cold war.

Once the cold war ended along with the end of the Soviet Union and the fall of the Berlin Wall, the American farmer was left with unprecedented debt, and no place to sell their crops. Then the banks foreclosed on the American farmers with no government to bail them out. Half of the big American wheat farmers disappeared. One farming-community in Montana took up arms against the United States in standoff lasting 81 days. The group called themselves the Freemen of Montana. (For further reading, go to: http://www.ipublishweb.com/ freemenstudy.html)

Regan was a president known as the President whose goal was to send a new image of prosperity. During his administration, the United States exposed the weaknesses of the Russian Communist Party and military during the Soviet invasion of Afghanistan. It ultimately ended a 20-year cold war, the end of the Soviet Union and the fall of the Berlin Wall.

There was also an assassination attempt on President Regan. He got shot but lived through the injury.

Regan left his Vice President George H. W. Bush with a great legacy, but soon President Bush had the country back in another war in the Persian Gulf called Desert Storm, but he never finished the job. He lost a second term in office thinking he was certain to win re-election. Arkansas Governor Bill Clinton campaigned furiously and won the presidency and a second term in office.

President Bill Clinton, on the other hand, kept us out of major wars and left the country with the best economy in my lifetime. Clinton also lost respect of the American people when he finally admitted to having an improper relationship with Monica Lewinsky, a young woman who worked in the White House. He is the one president who can look back and be proud of the way he ran the country economically. He left the country with a surplus of money and didn't drive us into any major wars.

After the Clinton administration ended, George W. Bush, the son of the first President Bush, became president. Then, all trust in government seemed to go downhill. About three months after he took office, terrorists attacked the United States by sending suicide operatives to fly two American passenger jets into the New York World Trade Center, one jet into the U.S. Pentagon and a fourth jet, Flight 93, believed to be targeting the White House. We were soon at war again against Afghanistan, a place where the religious extremists were training soldiers to make war against the West.

George W. Bush declared a second war in the Persian Gulf to end the reign of the deposed president of Iraq, Saddam Hussein, who was accused of war crimes and violating United Nations mandates. Rumors have it that because the Bush family had such huge oil interests in the Middle East, they got the United States into two major wars. The American economy nearly collapsed after his eight years in office.

Now President Barak Obama, who inherited the worst economy in my lifetime, seems to be seems to be trying, but I feel he made a mistake by bailing out the American banking industry. I think the money from the huge $700 billion stimulus package should have all gone to helping the American home owners save their homes instead of bailing out the banks. This way the economy would still be moving.

On immigration, it seems like it has gotten out of hand. For, instance the illegal Mexican population in America has grown ten times the size in the sixty years that I have been here. The problem isn't with the Mexican people, it is with illegal immigration. Last told, there was said to be 18 million undocumented Mexican immigrants in the United States.

Some of those illegals cross our border and bring drugs and crime. Their crimes include a problem of human trafficking. This is where American criminals capitalize on safe-houses and organized prostitution, and there is plenty of it going on all over most American cities.

The latest problem is on the topic of anchor babies—where illegals come to the United States while the women are pregnant. The children are born in the United States and are allowed to stay and go through our education system and get medical assistance through our welfare system. The problem with this is the parents often work for cash without paying taxes and Social Security. The honest immigrants and American citizens have to pay higher taxes and often times Social Security for these illegal actions. Right now, I believe there are probably more illegals collecting from our welfare assistance and Social Security fund than there are immigrants who pay into the system.

It is said that illegal immigration is driven by pressure of Americans not wanting to do the hard or hot jobs that don't pay well, but that isn't necessarily true, because I worked on shipping docks in 10 degrees below zero for almost a half year. Many Americans will do the jobs if the competition was not so fierce and they didn't have to compete with such low wages. A lot of these jobs are jobs that could be done by our kids during the summer months when school is out.

Often illegals come to America, and many of them live and share living expenses with ten other illegals bunking in the same house. Then, they take their money back to Mexico and support their families down there. That means the money they earn here does not go back into the American economy. This causes an imbalance.

I even have relations who do the same thing. They collect Social Security, pensions and wages earned here, and they take it and spend it all over Europe. The problem is millions of people and billions of dollars are leaving this country in this way, and it weakens our economy.

Even though Arizona has the controversial immigration law SB1070 which hurts some people in the short run. It might mean that taking on such measures is what it is going to take to turn this system around. Nobody wants to hurt people, but something has to be done before the system can't be fixed.

I also feel that the America needs to stop supporting the rest of the world without them paying us back or contributing to our society. They could contribute by buying things from us.

Another place to start changing is the politicians need to force laws to bring jobs back to America and put the workers back to work making products to sell overseas. We might have to place higher taxes on products that are made overseas and sold in America. Something has to put the American economy back on track. It's a vicious cycle because if they place too high of taxes on goods from overseas, then America could experience shortages here, which again drives the prices up through inflation.

One good example is when they opened up new JCPenney outlet in Goodyear, Arizona. I went into the store and met a salesman that grew up in Italy near my home in the Tenuta Neighborhood. After we met, we hit it off well just as friends from the old country. One day, I asked him if a jacket I liked went on sale to please call me and let me know. He did call and told me when the jacket went on sale. It was originally for sale at 209 dollars. I was able to buy it for 89 dollars. That means that there was a markup of 120 dollars. I suspect JCPenney could have sold it and made money at 89 dollars in the first place, but they are just set up to charge high prices and make big money instead of pricing items in the range for the normal person.

On top of that, the jacket was made in Taiwan and probably only cost JCPenney somewhere between 5 or 20 dollars in the first place.

As far as politicians go, I feel there should also be limits on how long politicians can serve. First of all, after a politician turns 65 years old, he or she should be ousted and younger politicians—who have up-to-date educations with fresh ideas—should be given a chance to run the country. The longer a politician is in office, the more power he or she has, and it is hard to get them out of office and let new people who are better-educated run the country. Even when they do leave office, the country has to continue to pay pensions that are sometimes just as high as their salaries and benefits for the rest of their lives and sometimes even their spouses. This has to change or we are going to have serious problems with cities, states and someday even the country not being able to keep up with paying pensions and benefits for people who already have enough money to live the rest of their life.

Another good example happened this year. The U.S. Government was almost forced to shut down. And if it had shut down, the politicians would still have received their pay, but the service men and women and their families would have received their paycheck late. This is wrong.

The politicians had from September to January to structure a new budget, but for political reasons, they waited until the last days of the year in order to cause pressure to get their own agendas passed. The amount in debate between the Democrat and Republican parties was 38 billion dollars. Instead of passing a budget, they wrote a temporary package into law. It will cost the taxpayer almost double to put the temporary package into law. It's a *damn* shame.

It should not be this way. They didn't do their job and they should be fired. Anyone else who doesn't do the job they are paid to do would get fired, but the politicians just do these things and continue to get away with it.

I heard a couple of weeks ago that our country is 15 trillion dollars in debt. Who is going to pay for that? Probably our grandchildren if it ever gets paid. If it doesn't get paid, then it's quite possible that some other country is going to run our country economically. China has already bought much of the American debt, so Americans are now paying interest payments to China and making China wealthy beyond belief. It is said that the United States is already paying millions of dollars per day in interest payments to China.

This is how I believe China has such a control over North Korea. I hate to see the same thing happen to parts of the United States where China one day controls sections of the country.

China now has over 2 billion people. I heard during the early 1970s China made a law restricting one child per family. Because there is such great honor in China to have sons, rather than daughters, it was told that the country evolved by the year 2000 to having more than 500 thousand war-aged male adults. That was double the entire population of the United States at the time. If we were to ever go to war with China, we could not win that war without major weapons mass destruction.

DOs & TABOOs

DO: *It is great to have different cultures here in the United States. As it says on the Statue of Liberty: Give me your tired, your poor, Your huddled masses yearning to breathe free.*

TABOO: *It is not so great to have millions of people here in the country working illegally, draining the economy, because it upsets the economic balance and any hope for a future of huddled masses yearning to breathe free.*

CHAPTER EIGHT

A Tribute To My Beloved Rosemary

From the first time I saw her, I thought Rosemary was the most precious young woman I had ever met. She was so beautiful that I had a hard time keeping my eyes off of her. I always thought that she resembled Sofia Loren, who at the time was one of the most glamorous women in films.

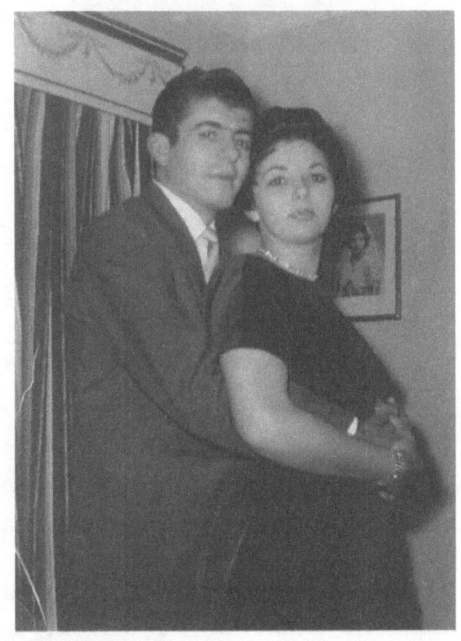

She had another trait that I adored: That trait was how committed she was to family. I knew from the very start that becoming close with her family was the only way I could ever get close to knowing her.

She was always so easy to please—beginning with the way we would spend Sundays together hanging out with her parents and playing Italian card games. When other young women would like running around, she was content to have me join her with her family like I was one of them. I liked the way she had respect for her parent's wishes. She was committed to her education and following the guidelines her parents set out for us when we went out on dates.

As we began seeing each other, she showed respect for her parents' wishes, and we didn't put ourselves into situations that could cause temptations—like when we went to my apartment, we only went to pick things up and left immediately—in order not to put ourselves in tempting situations.

Old school was a way of life for her including the day I proposed marriage. Asking me to ask her parents in a proper way was her first wish. In that way, she made it easy for me to be part of her family.

After dating for about six months, Rosemary got all dressed up for our date. She always dressed to the "Nines." She looked so nice that

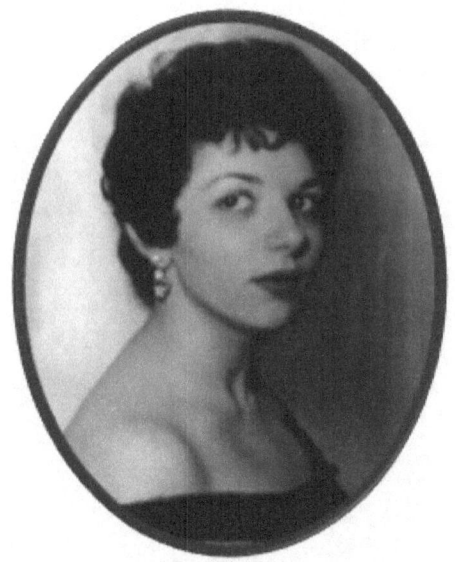

Adeline decided to take a picture of her in her beautiful dress. Right before she snapped the picture, I reached over and pulled Rosemary's blouse below her shoulders, which made a very seductive pose. To my surprise, Rosemary responded with a look of irritation. Adeline caught the picture capturing both the bare shoulders (considered too seductive in those days) and the stunned look of disapproval on her face.

Knowing how conservative Rosemary was in those days. The picture eventually became a family-favorite to all knew her—seeing a picture of her dressed seductively—without a smile on her face. Rosemary also came to appreciate the picture.

When Rosemary was still in high school, most of her close family members called her "Babe-Doll." Later, they dropped the word Doll off her name and called her "Babe." The name Babe stuck and stayed with her for her entire life—even when we later moved to Arizona in 1996, her cousins still called her Babe. The name even carried into the workplace.

Once, a friend of ours called her workplace and asked for Babe, The person who answered the phone asked: "Who is Babe?" Rosemary was sitting near to her and took the call, and from that day forward, she became known as Babe even where she worked at the Coldwell Banker Real Estate office. She was treated very well and was very well liked by all those around her. At Christmas time, she was always showered with gifts from her employers and coworkers. She always came out of work with a smile. Rosemary always looked forward to going to work and never complained about her job.

We just had a way of making fun times out of all of our experiences and the times we spent together. A lot of times, when I am all alone, I think about the things I would want to put in my book about Rosemary. It is so easy to say great and fun things about her.

She was such a good person.

She didn't have it in her personality to argue or even let people around her get upset. She seemed to know from her heart how to treat everyone with kindness. It was natural for her to calm me down when I would get excited. She always had faith that I shouldn't get excited because things would always work out. They always did work out.

Dressing up was important. When we went out on dates, we always dressed up classy. From our very first date to our 45-year wedding anniversary, she always had a charm that made me proud to be with her and made me feel like she was the most valuable person in my world.

Having her for a wife was like having the best support-person someone could ask for. We always knew where the other one was. She always knew when I was coming home and she would be there waiting for me when I got home from work. She would go the distance to make it possible for me to have special meals whenever I asked.

I loved her.

I loved the person I was when I was with her.

I loved marrying her.

I loved being married to her.

She had her ways of letting me know how much she loved being married to me. She was a good person, good woman, great wife and a tremendous mother. She was hard working, fun loving, smart, kind, honest and somehow I knew she was the perfect match for me.

We had a good friendship, a good marriage and a good relationship. She was in my life day and night. Night times, I still sit down and watch the television, and when I look at the bedroom door where she used to walk out after taking a shower, I remember how she always came out looking like a beautiful rose.

A good sense of humor is the best way to describe her personality. Sometimes I would comment how she looked so good. She would respond with a smile and then she would ask me to go get her some Ice cream. She loved ice cream. Her best trait was the way she always talked to me with a smile—even when things got tough.

On the thirteenth day of each month in 49 years of marriage, we celebrated another month of being together. The thirteenth day of each month was always treated as another anniversary. We made it a point to greet each other with hugs and kisses on these days. Of course, when it was our yearly anniversaries, I was always surprised with some type of little gift—even if it was just a small card. We often celebrated our anniversary by going out for another dinner date.

People enjoyed talking with her because of her ability to communicate well. It was just as important to her to let others know that they would be heard and understood.

When she played the organ, I liked to listen, but the sound of her music would often lull me to sleep because she played so beautiful. She would ask me if I wanted her to keep playing the organ or if I wanted to go back to sleep? I would always tell her that I wanted her to keep going. Even though she would look again and I would be dozing off again.

We went to Palm Springs for vacation from time to time. When we were there, she would look for little places to find bargains—looking for simple little gifts for me for the grandchildren. Once in a while she enjoyed buying herself little jewelry items.

Often times we went to yard sales or bargain shopping, it wasn't so much to buy something. It was just so we could go do something together. We enjoyed doing things together.

Rosemary was the best homemaker. The house came first. The home had to be clean—like spick and span. Most of the time, she was very casual about things. But when the kids were in school, she was very active in decisions about their school.

The children never missed a meal, and the meals were always home-cooking. When it was time for the children to go to bed, she was right there making the sure the kids were tucked in and getting their proper sleep. She always cooked special meals on Sundays.

Rosemary was always logical about saving money—even if it meant going to Mother's Day celebrations such as dinner the week before or the week after Mother's Day. It never bothered her.

On Mother's Day she often made Mother's Day dinners for her own mother. I loved cheese cake, and when I found out I am diabetic, she started creating me a sugar-free deserts. Nothing like that ever stopped her from pleasing me. When she was still cooking meals, my sugar levels were always stable. She always paid attention to my health—even after her own health started declining.

During times like Christmas and birthdays, we always asked each other what we had in our minds for gifts we wanted, and that is usually the way we bought each other presents. After we were married twenty five years, I gave her a card on our anniversary. It was a card with tickets for a vacation trip to Italy inside.

I always traded haircuts with other barbers in the area. Before we left for our trip to Italy, Barber Joe, who used to cut my hair, came to give me my regular haircut. As he clipped away, he asked: "What's up?"

I proceeded to explain: "I'm taking Rosemary for a vacation to Rome."

"ROME?!" Joe asked, "Why would you want to go there? It's a crowded dirty city full of the Mafioso! You'd be crazy to go to Rome! So, how are you getting there?"

"We're taking TWA," I replied.

"TWA?!" yelled Joe. "That's a terrible airline. Their planes are old, their flight attendants are ugly and they're always late! So where are you staying in Rome?"

I told him: "We'll be staying at the downtown International Marriot."

"That DUMP?" asked Joe. "That's the worst hotel in Rome! The rooms are small, the service is surly and slow and they're overpriced! So what are you going to do when you get there?"

I said: "We're going to go see the Vatican and hope to see the Pope."

"HA! That's rich!" laughs Joe. "Yah—you and a million other people trying to see him. He'll look the size of an ant. Boy, good luck on THIS trip. You're going to need it!"

Rosemary enjoyed the trip so much that we ended up going there four more times. She loved going to the souvenir shops at the Vatican. She loved to buy little jewelry for herself but mostly for our daughters-in-law and our granddaughters.

When anyone goes to the Roman Vatican, they are never allowed to move throughout the Vatican without an escort. When we went on tours, Rosemary was always so impressed by the church and being at the Vatican that she could sit for hours just looking and sometimes praying. Her favorite spot was the Sixteenth Chapel, which is the World of Arts. It seemed like she could sit and enjoy those things for long periods of time when they got her attention. It was usually me who would decide when it was time to leave. She really knew how to enjoy and appreciate those kinds of trips. She was the same way about marriage. For her it was more about being married than getting married. It was a commitment for life.

She was always so thankful about getting gifts like travel trips. She was grateful to have those memories, and she knew how to thank me in a way that I knew it really meant something special to her. She had a way of letting me know that she appreciated the trips, and more importantly, she appreciated that I had helped make the trips possible. She could get double the pleasure, by enjoying the trips and then giving the feelings of appreciation.

A month later, after we returned, Barber Joe came in for his regular haircut.

Joe asked: "Well, how did that trip to Rome turn out? I bet TWA gave you the worst flight of your life!"

"No, quite the opposite," I explained. "Not only were we on time in one of their brand new planes, but it was full so they bumped us up to first class. The food and wine were wonderful, and we had a beautiful 28-year-old flight attendant who waited on us hand and foot!"

"Hmmm," Joe said, "Well, I bet the hotel was just like I described."

"No, quite the opposite," I said. "They had just finished a 25-million dollar renovation. It's the finest hotel in Rome, now. They were overbooked, so they apologized and gave us the Presidential suite for no extra charge!"

"Well," Joe mumbled, "I *know* you didn't get to see the Pope!"

I told him: "Actually, we were quite lucky. As we toured the Vatican, a Swiss guard tapped Rosemary on the shoulder and explained the Pope likes to personally meet some of the visitors, and if we'd be so kind as to step into his private room and wait, the Pope would personally greet us. Sure enough, after 5 minutes the Pope walked through the door and shook our hands. We both knelt down as the Pope spoke a few words to me."

Impressed, Joe asked, "Tell me, please! What did he say?"

"Oh—not much really. Just 'Where'd I get my awful haircut?'" (Anonymous)

We renewed our wedding vows on our 45-year wedding anniversary. The whole event took place because I felt it was the right thing to do. The whole thing was a secret surprise for Rosemary.

I almost got caught, because right before the event took place, on Friday I went to pick up the children when they arrived from Chicago. The problem was that I was wearing shorts and I told Rosemary that I was going to work. When she saw the shorts she just said: "Give me another one—a tale."

She knew something was up, because she knew I never wore shorts to work. And when I got home, she opened the door to the garage, and there were all the children. She thought that was the big surprise. She still didn't know that the wedding vows event was coming on Sunday.

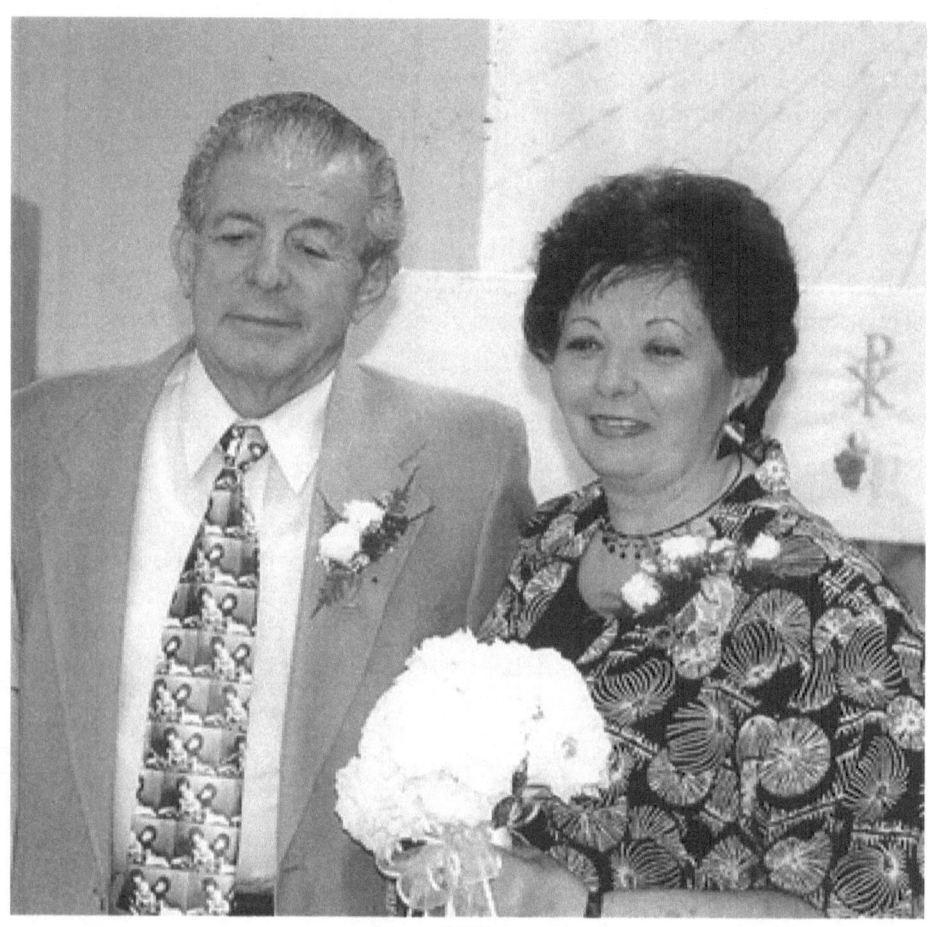

Without her knowing, I set up the whole thing ahead of time. I signed up for the time slot at St. Clare of Assisi Catholic Church. I made arrangements for the Priest to deliver the ceremony. I also made arrangements for the children and grandchildren to come to Arizona from Chicago to be part of our ceremony. I did my best to keep her from getting ahold of a church bulletin the week before. There was an announcement of the event in the bulletin.

We went to Mass on that Sunday, and she knew nothing about the surprise. Before Holy Communion, the Priest asked us to both come up to the Alter to renew our wedding vows. To Rosemary's surprise every one there knew it was taking place accept her. She was a little nervous when the Priest asked her if she knew anything about it. She said, "No." And with all the emotion, she had a few tears—especially when the congregation gave us a standing ovation.

Giving her big surprises was such a fun and important part of our relationship.

That day, Rosemary was just as charming as she was on the day we first married. I was also just as deeply in love and deeply committed at 45 years of marriage as I was the day we married.

Now that she has passed, people tell me that time will heal. In my case, the pain is still there and it doesn't seem to get any better as time goes on. Sometimes I go on walks and if someone asks me where I am going, I say well, I don't know where I am going, but I will let you know when I get back. She is what I really want and she is not here anymore. When I go on walks my mind seems to travel back in time to a place where I feel the joy from my memories. It helps me to survive. I guess losing Rosemary is what the Good Lord decided is best, and it's what I have to accept. If she were looking down—seeing me going through this pain—she would just say: "Things will get better, so do the best with what you have." And, I know, even from above, she would tell me this with a smile.

CHAPTER NINE

Family Values

This chapter is devoted to ideas I have about family values. With this chapter, I hope to touch deep into the hearts and souls of my family, my friends and anyone who reads *Life of A Barber—The DOs & TABOOs*

Each earlier chapter mentioned events in my life as a barber. Up to this point, at the end of most chapters, there were *DOs & TABOOs* sections noted. But here in this chapter, you will read strings of *DOs & TABOOs* throughout the chapter as I need to stress the importance of my family values.

Reiterated Definitions:

DO—An action or thought proscribed by society as proper or acceptable to execute.

TABOO—An action or thought proscribed by society as improper or unacceptable. (Dictionary.com)

As I mentioned earlier, as far as I can remember, no stories were ever told. No stories were written—that I can say were handed down over the generations about the long history and tradition of the Tenuta Family. I also never found a book that explains the sure way raise my children in a perfect way to encourage family values.

In this chapter, you will read things that were confusing to me and things that might seem confusing to you. By telling you my honest thoughts with the use of *DOs & TABOOs*, I hope to create a family legacy (this book) bound with love, hope and dreams of a future.

I don't want to be remembered as a grumpy old man who died full of pain and disappoint during the last years of my life. I do, however feel it is important to be truthful and mention things which took place with my family members that felt very hurtful.

I apologize in advance if things I mention—which are personal and family in nature—hurt or offend anyone who reads this book. But, this is a chapter in my life. I feel if I were to leave it out of the book, then the purpose of my life—promoting family values—would never get passed on.

To begin, let me mention that my success is measured in many ways. For the most part, I measured success by my own set of standards. So, defining success is in large part about expectations I have set. Right or wrong, I am willing to look at my part to see which expectations are real and which are too high.

My 49 years with Rosemary was like a dream-come-true. Looking back, the time came and went so fast. The last 3-1/2 years seemed like hell on earth—seeing her suffer with her illness.

It is not my intent to only bring out hurtful memories, but also to provide advice in hopes that much of the joy that Rosemary and I shared can be salvaged and passed on in matters that really count when it comes to my family, friends and others.

One thing I want to say here is that I understand that everyone deals with death and funerals in their own way. There really is no correct way to handle death and loss. But for some people, with each loss, there can be a period of feeling alone and confused. I was no different.

I understand that each one of us owes a death. There are no exceptions. The further I am from the loss of Rosemary, means the closer to my own end. The true meaning of family values seems to get clearer and more urgent as time passes.

I feel that my age gives me the privilege of giving advice and providing guidance to my sons and other family members. So, I hope they read this chapter and follow it through to its end. Hopefully, in some little way, my advice will steer them onto a course of peace, goodwill and forgiveness.

The loss of Rosemary is the hardest thing I ever could ever imagine experiencing. We had always planned that it would be the opposite—that I would probably be the first to pass away. She and I prepared our life and finances around that idea. It was not so. Instead, Rosemary was sickened by kidney disease and liver failure. Our whole world was turned up-side-down. It is clear that the pain I experienced and continue to feel was nothing compared to the slow tortuous end she met.

The next hardest thing I have ever experienced is my confusion about my sons having such a distance between them.

I feel it would be a great success if somehow I could get through to Robert and John and have them join together and help me find a way to pull this family back together. It would be another dream come true—not an expectation.

Mentioning their hostility is not for gaining pity, but rather to open their eyes to a layer of family values that could bring so much joy to me, their children and most importantly to themselves. Rosemary and I always hoped for something different and stronger between them. Any parents would love to see their kids be bound together.

We would have moved the heavens and earth to see Robert and John love and cherish each other—like Rosemary and I cherished each other. It is not so. Not as brothers growing together, not as family bonded with the love, hope and dreams of a future, not as the generations of the Tenuta family that stretches across the globe from the motherland of Italy to sunny Arizona, but as enemies.

Rosemary is gone, so it's too late to heal any wounds she suffered as a result of the rivalry that pitted her sons against each other. Perhaps it's getting too late for me to see the joy of my sons bonded in humor and hopes of a future.

However, it is not too late to come together in a generous way, which can only enrich the souls of my precious grandchildren.

Most importantly, one of the life's greatest treasures is to have a brother. Having a brother is something that will never change. Moreover, having a brother who is close can be one of the most valuable experiences.

I often thought: "If only for Rosemary's sake, maybe the boys could find a way to come together." But that is not right. In a small selfish way, I would love to see our boys overcome their rivalry for my sake. But that is not the right reason either. There are even times when I feel terrible about the loss that my grandchildren have experienced as a result of their rivalry. Even that is not the right reason for them to come together. Neither Rosemary's hurt, nor my pain, nor the grandchildren's losses can even start to compare to damage caused by their own lost opportunity of enjoying each other.

I was once told that two people working together can accomplish more than three people working separately. With this in mind, I imagine how strong my two sons could be working together, just as their two wives working together, just as their six grandchildren working together—even if they only worked together for the enjoyment and fulfillment of a big family.

It is not so.

An enemy is how Robert treats his brother John. Where harsh words feel like knives and his silent anger cripples any chance for my grandchildren being strengthened by the yoke of family values and the fulfilling pride of their long life-line which has survived the worst imaginable poverty and ravages of a world war.

The harshness that Robert feels for John continues to this day. Even their children seem to be pitted against each other, where Robert won't even open up a chance for my grandchildren to get to know each other and form their own relationships.

It's a selfish **TABOO**

It all started when the boys were young. Robert and John would come home from school and Robert would pick on John. Rosemary and I finally reached a point that we were forced to ask a neighbor to watch over John until we got home from work, because for the lack of a better word, Robert would "crucify" John. When Robert was alone with John, he would bully him and taunt him so much that we feared what might happen to John if we didn't do something to protect him. This behavior ultimately continued right up to the end of Rosemary's life. Nearly forty years since it all started, the ill-feelings that Robert carries for John still seem to be ongoing. Rosemary and I were both left feeling hopeless and broken-hearted.

When Rosemary died in Orland Park, the whole family was there at her wake. But she wanted to be buried in Arizona, so I offered to pay the expense of flying Robert to Arizona for her funeral. Soon after, some of the worst imaginable things happened.

Robert said he would come to Arizona to attend Rosemary's funeral, so I thought the least I could do is offer to pay for his plane ticket. I also offered to let him stay in our master bedroom while he was visiting.

Aside from the fact that Robert didn't even try to be courteous enough to attempt to get a bereavement airfare, which would have helped—considering all the extra expenses of the funeral. The saddest thing was that he came with one suitcase full of his own clothing for the trip, but while he was here, he packed up two additional suitcases full of Rosemary's personal-belongings and took them from my home.

I wonder how many people would see what he did as a low-class **TABOO**.

Those personal belongings included all of her valuable jewelry and all of her life-long treasures, which by all rights should have been divided among all the heirs by me.

That was the right thing to **DO**

Robert decided he would take it upon himself to keep it all. It never crossed my mind that he would do such a thing. At that time, I was in no place emotionally to be watching what he was doing in our bedroom.

I was sleeping in the guest room because I had promised Rosemary that I would not sleep in our bedroom until she returned from Chicago, and all of her medical was finished.

Early on, Rosemary and I could only guess that Robert's behavior was maybe out of jealousy of having a younger sibling. But now it seems to be deeper than that. It seems Robert prefers to have distance between him and his brother and perhaps even between me. Even up until today, if I mention anything about John to Robert, his anger hits the roof.

*It has gone past **TABOO***

I feel that Robert really never wanted John as his brother. Robert acted as though he wanted his parents all to himself. We finally decided that when John was born, Robert had to share his parents with his younger brother, and that is why he didn't want anything to do with John. Robert's wife Monica said she agrees that Robert wanted his parents all to himself. Robert always acted as if he felt we treated John more favorable than him.

John is also my son and regardless of how Robert feels about having John for a brother.

*John is a **DO**!*

Our friend, Father Bill Finnegan, knew what was going on between the boys. When the Father saw Robert at the church, he approached Robert to talk with him about it, but Robert gave the Priest the same cold shoulder. After mass, the Priest told me there was no way of getting through to Robert. He said: "Robert is hard to reach." He suggested that we just do the best with what we have.

*How do you do the best you can with a **TABOO**?*

I wish Robert would seek help about the rivalry he carries, even if it is with someone other than Father Finnegan, who Robert has known for more than ten years. If Robert would just get some guidance from someone who he could confide in and trust, then he could understand what he is doing to others around him—and more importantly—what he is doing to himself. Hopefully, he would stop the vicious cycle of torment which could eventually get passed on to his own precious children.

That would be a **DO**

I feel it is partly my responsibility to bring these things to light. After all, saving my grandchildren is one of the reasons I am bringing this issue out into the open in this book. Hopefully, if he reads this and tries to understand the torment his mother experienced and that I am experiencing, then he might try to change things for the better and possibly save his own children from the same fate.

As far as Robert goes, I don't understand; the people he likes, he will go all out for them. But, if he doesn't like someone, he won't have anything to do with them. He has very nice neighbors. One neighbor lives next door and the other lives around the corner. Our family has known them for years. Robert has nothing to do with them.

That's a real **TABOO**

I think what Robert needs, like what all of us need, is a good sense of humor. John and I were once talking about a movie we both watched named: *Two Faces of Evil* with Joanne Woodward and Paul Newman. The movie suggests the same idea about the need for a sense of humor. In the movie, when Woodward likes someone, she was good to them, but when she didn't like them, she was just the way I describe Robert—Rude!

Let me say here that dealing with Robert in matters like this is like walking with two feet in one shoe.

Once, our long-time neighbor friends from Orland Park were visiting Las Vegas. They called my son John and invited him to come join them. John went and was happy to see them. They paid for John's whole trip. The tab was picked up entirely by them. The hotel, food and the trip—everything was paid. They told John: "We want you here. We want you to feel like our guest." It was such a good gesture on their part.

That was very fine example of a **DO**

I also went to see the same neighbors in Orland Park, and they took me out to lunch. Everything was complete. They are such nice people. They are people from the old neighborhood who we have known for nearly 35 years.

Those friends just **DO** *and* **DO** *and* **DO**

Robert doesn't want to have anything to do with them. I don't think the way Robert acts to them is something we taught in our family. We all considered each other friends, and we all respected one another. Robert is just different in that way.

If Robert doesn't like a person, then he doesn't have to insult them. He doesn't have to hurt their feelings. He could just say "Hello or goodbye—or something—and let it go at that. He doesn't have to treat them rude, but he does.

That's **TABOO**

My son John remarked that: "Someday, something not so good could happen to Robert, and our old friends in the neighborhood—that Robert has treated this way could just say: 'To Hell with Him.'" But they probably would help him anyway. I feel that there could come a time when he needs people like them—neighbors who could help him in return for the kindness he has shown to them.

There would be nothing more pleasurable for me than to have seen my sons come together. Unfortunately we never got to enjoy seeing a communion between them; instead, we always experienced the fear of the way they were going to act with each other. It seems to be entirely Robert's choice to be on the "outs" with John. It would be my final wish for him to become a loving brother to John.

That would be a **DO**

John has always, to my knowledge tried to become closer and friendlier to Robert, but Robert, to this day won't accept his friendship.

John has been much different than Robert—trying to at least to try to make something work between the two of them. He is also different and kinder to people. Up until a few years ago, John seemed to do the right things. Whenever he saw Robert, he would shake his hand.

But now he seems to have just given up on changing Robert.

I would love to see all my grandchildren get a chance to come to know each other on a greater level and experience the love and passion that cousins deserve to have with each other, which has been wrongfully taken from them by Robert.

In response to this, a year after Rosemary passed away, the only words Robert left us with was: "The person that I loved is gone now, and to hell with the rest of you."

That was a cruel **TABOO**

As for John, I just wish he would have listened to me from day one a little closer in matters of business and money. I believe he could be a millionaire with the kind of food he serves at his restaurants. I think with an open mind and taking more of my advice, he could have avoided some of the financial hardships he has experienced. I would like to see him focus more on advertising. It is one of the keys to success in business. Perhaps his shortcomings in business are driven in part by budget, but sometimes I think there is stubbornness in him which holds him back. I feel he is listening now, and he will take more of my advice in such matters.

That's a **DO**

If he would just listen to the old man in these matters, then he could begin to rebuild his reputation and have a great and prosperous future. Experience is the best teacher. And I think my experience in business is the best he could possibly get.

There was a time when Christina went to Chicago to visit Rosemary in Orland Park. Monica seemed resentful that Christina came unannounced. I never understood Monica's resentments. Monica seems much like Robert in those ways.

That was **TABOO**

But on the other hand, Monica really stepped up big during the last 1-1/2 years of Rosemary's life. She helped Rosemary with her medical problems sometimes every day until she died. And for that I am deeply grateful. And for her effort, she was compensated the best way I could. During that time, Monica took Rosemary to her dialysis treatments four times per week for the whole time. I am so grateful to her for what she did for Rosemary. I feel total joy over the way Monica helped Rosemary in the end.

That was her biggest DO

I tried to explain to Rosemary that Robert and Monica don't seem to want to see their children get together with John's and Christina's children. I have the feeling that my grandchildren in Chicago, who are young now, will likely grow up to be just like Robert and Monica and ignore their parents. I hope not, but kids usually say and do the things they see their parents say and do.

My grandchildren in Arizona would like to see their cousins and be closer, but because of Robert and Monica, it probably won't happen unless it happens later in life after their childhood is gone and it's too late to be kids together.

One time, I wanted a picture of my six grandchildren together. The way I had to get a picture of all six grandchildren in one picture was to take a picture of Robert's three children, and then, I took another picture of John's three children. I brought both pictures to the photo shop and had Hallmark put the two pictures together. It destroys me to see the same kind of separation among my grandchildren.

It was by mere chance one day when John's wife, Christina, was driving through the neighborhood in Orland Park. She saw Robert's three children playing together in their front yard. Because Christina had her and John's own three children with her in the car, she seized the moment. She had the foresight to stop her car, and she got her three children out and pulled all six of our grandchildren together to get a picture of all six children in the same photo. That was a real blessing for us—to see all of our six grandchildren together.

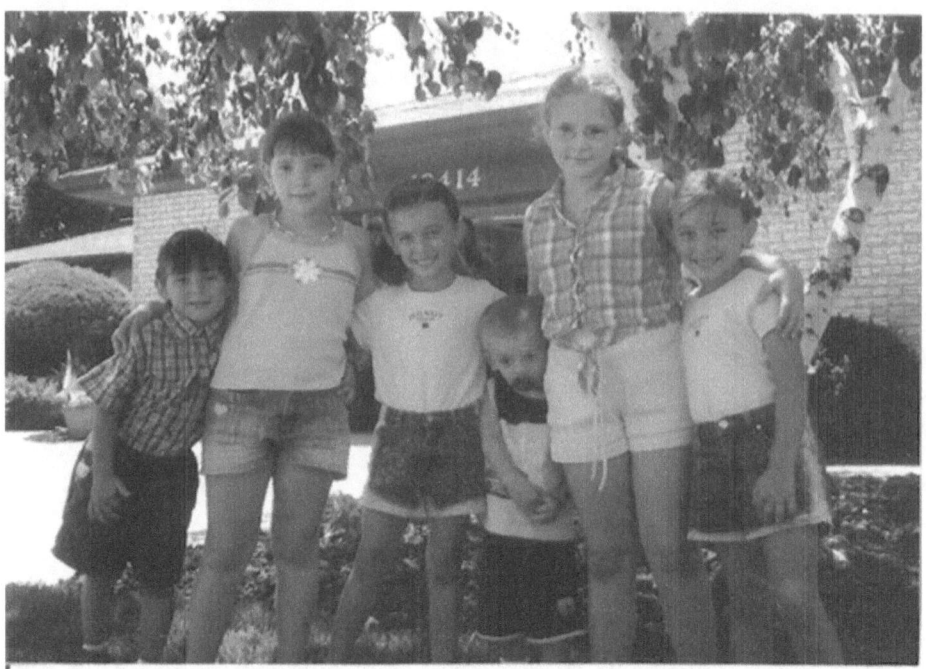

It is such a blessing to have this picture of all my grandchilren together. I praise Christina for having the foresight to see how much it means to me--and of course my beloved Rosemary. I thank you from the bottom of my heart.

That is my all-time favorite **DO***.*

I am not sure what Robert hopes to gain by keeping the grandchildren apart, but it sure caused a lot of disappointment for me and for Rosemary.

As I mentioned earlier in the book, there was a man, Julius Hinton, who became a very good friend of the neighborhood. He came to Rosemary's wake, and he was the last person to leave. He was there to give me such kind support.

That was a caring and respectful **DO**

Earlier, I mentioned that two people working together can accomplish more than three people working separately. It would be great to see my boys working together, their wives working together and my grandchildren working together. The same effort can apply if my family would use (1) their education with (2) our family values to create a new tradition of today that could be passed on to many generations like the traditions from the motherland which brought us to today.

That would be a **DO**

One relative of ours, a cousin of Robert's would come to see the kids during the holidays and bring them gifts, but she didn't even have the courtesy of walking up the stairs to wish Rosemary well or give her seasons-greetings. Robert and his cousin are *"Two of a Kind."* She too is educated. God help the America education system if it only gets used for self-serving purposes. If you have a great education and on the other hand you forget family values, then what good is the education?

TABOO

Also, when Rosemary was sick, neither Lucy, Fred's wife, nor her kids (all educated) called Rosemary—even once. What happened to the family values?

When Rosemary died, they didn't even come to the wake. There was no respect shown to her. Now when I get a Christmas card from them, it is hard for me to forget the way they treated her. At times I felt like throwing it way.

Lucy was a school teacher. I think education is great if a person uses it for the right things. One of Lucy's son's was a dentist. With all that education, it seems like they could have figured out to come see Rosemary or to show support to our family during the time of our loss. Neither of them even came to the wake when she died. I am not alone in these feelings. My son John saw the same disrespect and told me he feels the same way. I feel ashamed about those people who fail to use God's gift of education in the right way.

That was **TABOO!**

On the other hand, there's Joe Ruffolo, who was born in America, but was a descendent of the Ruffolo neighborhood in Italy. He became pals with my brother Fred. They met in Kenosha a couple years after my brother came to America. After Joe found out Rosemary was sick, he always called her at least once per month. Even until this day, he continues our friendship and continues to call me to stay in touch. He was the only one from Kenosha who called when Rosemary got sick.

That was a sincere **DO**

Now, I go for walks and people ask me where I am going. I just tell them: "I'll let you know when I return." The thing I get from the long walks is remembering how Rosemary was a good companion—always with a smile. I know deep down she wants me to be happy. But things that have happened since losing her make it very hard. At times, I feel in by losing her, I lost a large part of myself. The behavior from Robert and those other relatives seems to intensify the hurt.

Today, almost three years later, I still sleep in the guest bedroom, because I still can't get myself together enough to go sleep in our room without her there. When I do go in the bedroom, I still picture Rosemary there, and it still brings up too many sad memories. What keeps me going now are the good memories that I have from the time she was here with me.

To sum this all up, I have decided to go by the wise words that Rosemary told me so many times: "Just do the best with what I have. Things will work out."

Being a man of faith, I have to believe her words are true. As I look for answers on how to deal with the struggle I go through with the rivalry between my sons, the answers I get seem to be telling me that I have to accept Robert for who he has become and let him go through whatever comes from the hurt and damage he is causing. I must believe that God would forgive him for what he is doing.

Along this line, I have to ask myself two questions:

If God is the head of my life and values, then how would my Heavenly Father have me deal with this?

If God can forgive him, "What makes me so almighty that I cannot?

Therefore, I believe if I am going to teach Robert the real strength that can come from family values and forgiveness, then I should find a way to be the first to forgive.

*That will be my **DO**.*

In closing, I was recently talking with a customer about the pain I continue to feel over my loss of Rosemary.

While I was cutting his hair, he reminded me of my faith.

He said: "John, God created the Heavens and the Earth in six days, right?"

"Right, I said."

He said: "John, when Jesus rose on Easter, he told his disciples: In my Father's house are many mansions . . . . and I go to prepare a place for you. (John: 14: 2)

"So John, if Jesus left this world to prepare a place for you in his Father's house where there are many mansions," he asked: "Then, what kind of place is he preparing for you that has taken Him 2011 years to **DO**?"

And why did he call Rosemary early to help him?"

"John," he said, "I don't have all your answers, but I can assure you of two things:"

(1) "They are **DO**-ing something really great;" and,

(2) "Rosemary is **DO**-ing it with a mile-long smile." (G.M.)

God Bless everyone who reads this book. John Tenuta

End